DARK FE

ENERGY

Say Goodbye to Peer Pressure and Unrealistic Standards, Unleash Your Inner Femme Fatale, Learn to Set Your Own Rules, Ignite Your Self-Confidence and Seduce with Your Magnetism

CATHERINE STONE

Table of Contents

INTRODUCTION: DEVELOP AND GROW THE POWER OF YOUR DARK FEMININE ENERGY 5

CHAPTER 1: BREAK FREE FROM PEER PRESSURE: BE YOUR AUTHENTIC SELF 8

How Society's Unrealistic Standards and Peer Pressure Are Influencing You 8

How to Embrace Individuality and Uniqueness 12

The Fundamentals of Self-Acceptance and Self-Love .. 18

CHAPTER 2: EMBRACING SENSUALITY AND FEMININE POWER 31

Get to Know the Archetype of the Femme Fatale 31

How to Be Sensual and How to Free Yourself from Sexual Bias, You Can Say Goodbye to Shame 36

Unleash the Power of Emotional Intelligence and Enhance Intuition 39

CHAPTER 3: SET YOUR OWN RULES: FIND OUT HOW TO DEFY EXPECTATIONS AND CREATE YOUR OWN PATH 46

FREE YOURSELF FROM GENDER ROLES AND STEREOTYPES 46

FIND OUT WHICH ARE YOUR VALUES AND BELIEFS 56

HOW TO ESTABLISH BOUNDARIES AND ASSERT YOURSELF 59

CHAPTER 4: IGNITE SELF-CONFIDENCE: EMBRACE YOUR STRENGTHS AND OVERCOME LIMITATIONS . 68

SAY GOODBYE TO SELF-DOUBT AND START CULTIVATING INNER CONFIDENCE 68

Overcoming Self-Doubt 72

PAINT YOUR POSITIVE SELF-IMAGE AND EMBRACE BODY CONFIDENCE 78

HOW TO OVERCOME FAILURES AND LEARN FROM LIFE'S CHALLENGES 82

CHAPTER 5: SEDUCTION AND MAGNETISM: THE CHARISMATIC PRESENCE WAY 89

FIND OUT YOUR UNIQUE CHARMS AND AUTHENTICITY 89

BOOST YOUR COMMUNICATION AND SOCIAL SKILLS 95

Developing Effective Communication Skills 96

Enhancing Social Skills 100

BASICS OF MAGNETIC PRESENCE AND ATTRACTING POSITIVE CONNECTIONS 105

CHAPTER 6: THE ART OF SEDUCTION: MASTERING THE POWER TO CAPTIVATE MEN 110

A JOURNEY INTO THE PSYCHOLOGY OF MALE ATTRACTION ... 110

RELEASE YOUR SEDUCTIVE ENERGY AND CHARISMA 115

HOW TO NURTURE EMOTIONAL CONNECTION AND BUILD INTIMACY 122

CONCLUSION: INTEGRATE YOUR DARK FEMININE ENERGY 129

Introduction: Develop and Grow the Power of Your Dark Feminine Energy

In a world that often celebrates light, positivity, and harmony, it is easy to overlook the immense power and wisdom that lies within our darker aspects. The concept of the Dark Feminine Energy offers a compelling perspective on embracing the shadowy depths of our being, empowering us to tap into a wellspring of strength, transformation, and self-discovery.

This exploration does not imply promoting negativity, destructive tendencies, or harming others. Rather, it calls for a deeper understanding and acceptance of the aspects of ourselves that are typically marginalized or repressed. By acknowledging and embracing these facets, we gain access to a wellspring of profound wisdom, creativity, and personal growth.

Society has long imposed limitations on women, dictating what is acceptable and desirable. The dark feminine energy challenges these societal constructs and empowers women to reclaim their authentic selves, free from the expectations and constraints of others. It encourages a deep exploration of the self, embracing both the light and the shadows that reside within us.

By developing and growing the power of your dark feminine energy, you embark on a path of self-discovery, self-acceptance, and self-empowerment. It is an invitation to embrace the full spectrum of who you are, honoring every aspect of your being, including the parts that have been overlooked, suppressed, or deemed unworthy.

Throughout this journey, you will delve into the depths of your emotions, unraveling the threads that have woven your past experiences and conditioning. You will learn to navigate the complexities of your own psyche, shedding light on the shadows and integrating them into a harmonious whole.

In this exploration, you will find the strength to stand firmly in your truth, unapologetically embracing your desires, passions, and ambitions. The dark feminine energy ignites a fire within, propelling you forward with courage, resilience, and a fierce determination to create the life you envision.

This book is designed to assist you in developing and growing the power of your dark feminine energy. It will provide insights, tools, and practices that support your journey of self-discovery, healing, and empowerment. As you navigate this transformative path, remember that the dark feminine energy is not something to conquer or suppress; it is a force to be harnessed, respected, and integrated into the tapestry of your existence.

May this exploration of the dark feminine energy lead you to embrace your authentic power, reconnect with your inner wisdom, and shine your unique light in the world.

Let us embark on this enlightening odyssey together.

Chapter 1:

Break Free from Peer Pressure: Be Your Authentic Self

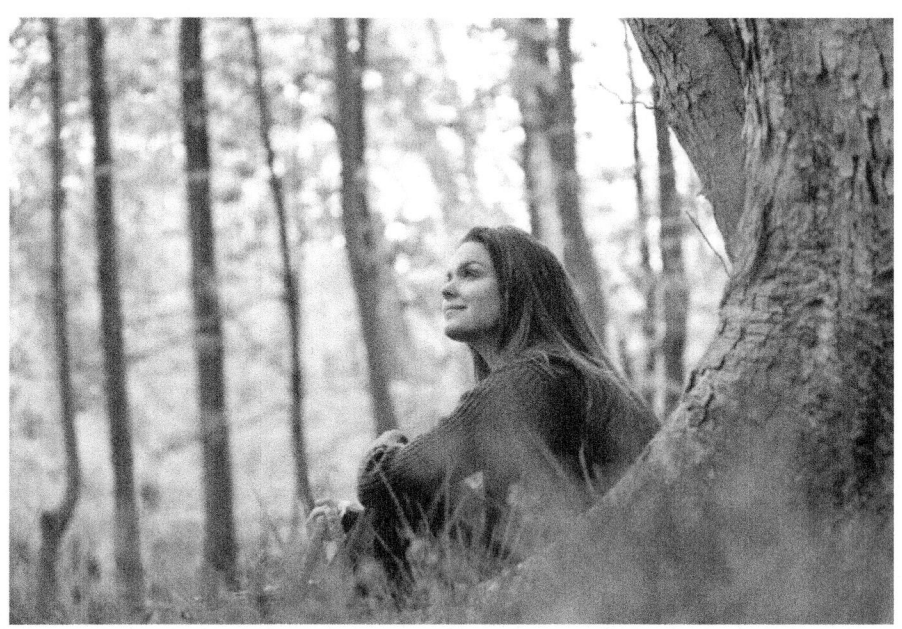

How Society's Unrealistic Standards and Peer Pressure Are Influencing You

As a woman, society's unrealistic standards and peer pressure can have a significant influence on various aspects of life, including appearance, behavior, career choices, and personal relationships. These influences can shape a woman's self-perception, confidence, and overall well-being.

One of the most prominent areas where unrealistic standards affect women is in terms of physical appearance. Society often promotes narrow definitions of beauty that are often unattainable and unrealistic. The media, advertising, and social platforms frequently portray airbrushed and heavily edited images, creating an unattainable standard of beauty that many women feel pressured to conform to. This may result in unhappiness with one's appearance, a lack of self-esteem, and possibly problems with one's mental health like eating disorders and depression.

Moreover, unrealistic standards extend beyond physical appearance and seep into various other aspects of a woman's life. Women often face pressure to conform to specific gender roles and expectations, such as being nurturing, submissive, or self-sacrificing. These expectations can limit their choices and opportunities, hindering their personal and professional growth. Additionally, women may face societal pressure to balance multiple roles, such as being a successful career woman, a devoted partner, and a nurturing mother, often feeling overwhelmed and judged when they are unable to meet all of these expectations simultaneously.

Peer pressure also plays a significant role in shaping a woman's behavior and choices. Women may face pressure from friends, colleagues, or family members to conform to certain societal norms or expectations. For example, they might feel pressured to conform to specific dress codes, engage in particular hobbies or interests, or make certain life choices, such as marriage or having children, based on their peers' expectations. This pressure can create a sense of conformity and limit a woman's ability to express her individuality and make choices that align with her true desires and aspirations.

The influence of society's unrealistic standards and peer pressure can also affect women's career choices and professional aspirations. Women may face societal expectations to pursue traditionally feminine or caregiving roles, which can deter them from entering male-dominated fields or pursuing ambitious career paths. Stereotypes and biases can also lead to unequal opportunities, pay gaps, and limited representation for women in leadership positions. These factors contribute to a lack of diversity and reinforce gender inequalities within the workplace.

Personal relationships can also be influenced by societal standards and peer pressure. Women may feel pressured to conform to societal expectations of romantic relationships, such as finding a partner by a certain age or adhering to traditional gender roles within the relationship. These pressures can impact a woman's decisions regarding dating, marriage, and starting a family. They may feel judged or stigmatized if they deviate from these norms, leading to feelings of inadequacy or fear of being perceived as "different."

It is important to recognize and challenge these unrealistic standards and peer pressure that women face. Promoting diverse representations of beauty, advocating for equal opportunities in all spheres of life, and encouraging individuality and authenticity can help combat these influences. Additionally, fostering supportive and inclusive environments where women can express themselves without fear of judgment is crucial. By challenging societal expectations and embracing individuality, women can lead fulfilling lives on their own terms, free from the constraints of unrealistic standards and peer pressure.

How to Embrace Individuality and Uniqueness

In a society that often promotes conformity and adhering to social norms, embracing our individuality can be a transformative act of self-love and self-acceptance. Listed below are various strategies and practices that can help us embrace our individuality and uniqueness.

1. Self-Reflection

Embracing individuality begins with self-reflection. Take the time to explore your values, interests, passions, and strengths. Reflect on what truly matters to you and what brings you joy. Self-reflection allows you to gain a deeper understanding of yourself, your desires, and your goals. It helps you identify the unique qualities and attributes that make you who you are.

2. Acceptance and Self-Love

Embracing individuality requires accepting and loving yourself unconditionally. Recognize that you are worthy and deserving of love and respect, just as you are. Embrace your strengths, but also accept your flaws and imperfections. Develop the habit of practicing self-compassion, where you consistently show yourself kindness and understanding. Foster a constructive and supportive connection with your own being, focusing on promoting positivity and personal growth.

3. Authenticity

Embracing individuality means being true to yourself and living authentically. It involves aligning your actions, choices, and behaviors with your inner values and beliefs. Embrace your unique perspectives and opinions, even if they differ from societal norms or expectations. Avoid pretending to be someone you're not or conforming to please others. Authenticity attracts genuine connections and allows you to live a life that is true to your essence.

4. Embrace Your Passions and Talents

Discover and embrace your passions and talents. Engage in activities that bring you fulfillment and joy, regardless of what others may think. Whether it's painting, writing, singing, or playing a musical instrument, allow your passions to shine and dedicate time to nurturing them. Embracing your talents and pursuing your passions not only brings you personal satisfaction but also helps you express your unique voice and gifts to the world.

5. Challenge Limiting Beliefs

Often, we hold limiting beliefs about ourselves that hinder our ability to embrace our individuality. These beliefs may be rooted in fear, self-doubt, or external judgments. Identify these limiting beliefs and challenge them. Replace them with positive and empowering beliefs that support your individuality and uniqueness. Surround yourself with individuals who uplift and encourage you to be your authentic self.

6. Cultivate a Supportive Environment

Surround yourself with a supportive community that celebrates and embraces individuality. Seek out like-minded individuals who appreciate and encourage diversity. Engage in open and honest conversations where you can express your thoughts and ideas without fear of judgment. Create a safe space where you can be yourself, free from societal pressures and expectations.

7. Practice Self-Expression

Find creative ways to express yourself and communicate your unique identity. This could involve various forms of self-expression, such as art, fashion, writing, or even public speaking. Experiment with different modes of self-expression that resonate with you. Allow yourself to be vulnerable and share your authentic self with others. Remember that self-expression is a powerful tool for connecting with others who appreciate and resonate with your uniqueness.

8. Embrace Difference

Embracing your individuality also involves embracing the individuality of others. Celebrate diversity and appreciate the unique qualities and perspectives that each person brings. Recognize that differences enrich our lives and broaden our understanding of the world. Engaging with diverse communities and learning from different cultures and experiences can expand your own sense of self and help you appreciate the beauty of individuality.

9. Practice Mindfulness

Cultivate mindfulness to stay present and connected with your authentic self. Mindfulness enables you to observe your thoughts and emotions without judgment, enabling you to connect with your true essence. Set aside time for meditation, deep breathing exercises, or any other mindfulness practices that resonate with you. By being present and mindful, you can tap into your inner wisdom and intuition, making choices that align with your authentic self.

10. Embrace Growth and Change

Embracing individuality is an ongoing process of growth and self-discovery. Be open to change and allow yourself to evolve over time. Embrace new experiences, step out of your comfort zone, and be willing to challenge yourself. Recognize that personal growth often involves embracing unfamiliar territory and embracing the unknown. Trust in your ability to adapt and grow as you continue to discover new aspects of your individuality.

11. Set Boundaries

Establishing boundaries is essential for embracing individuality. Clearly communicate your needs, values, and limits to others. Learn to say no to situations or people that compromise your authentic self. Setting boundaries ensures that you prioritize your well-being and protect your individuality from external pressures or expectations.

12. Practice Self-Compassion

Embracing individuality can be challenging at times, especially when faced with societal pressures or criticism. Practice self-compassion by treating yourself with understanding, kindness, and forgiveness. Acknowledge that everyone makes mistakes and that it's okay to stumble along the way. Offer yourself the same compassion and understanding you would give to a dear friend.

13. Seek Inspiration

Surround yourself with sources of inspiration that celebrate individuality. Seek out books, movies, art, and other forms of media that portray diverse perspectives and celebrate uniqueness. Engage with individuals who have embraced their individuality and learn from their journeys. Draw inspiration from those who have overcome societal expectations and achieved greatness by staying true to themselves.

14. Practice Gratitude

Cultivate a sense of gratitude for the uniqueness and individuality that you possess. Appreciate the qualities, experiences, and opportunities that have shaped you into the person you are today. Gratitude helps shift your focus towards the positive aspects of your individuality, fostering self-acceptance and a deeper sense of fulfillment.

15. Reflect and Adjust

Regularly reflect on your journey of embracing individuality. Assess what aspects of your life feel aligned with your authentic self and what areas may still need attention. Be open to making adjustments and course corrections along the way. Embracing individuality is not a linear path but a continuous process of self-discovery and growth.

The Fundamentals of Self-Acceptance and Self-Love

In your journey towards self-discovery and personal growth, the fundamentals of self-acceptance and self-love play a vital role. It is essential to develop a strong sense of acceptance and love for yourself, embracing your unique qualities, strengths, and imperfections. This section delves into the fundamentals of self-acceptance and self-love, providing practical strategies to foster these qualities in your life.

Embrace Your Uniqueness

Take a moment to appreciate the qualities that make you unique. Recognize that you are one-of-a-kind, with a combination of talents, interests, and experiences that set you apart from others. Embracing your uniqueness allows you to value yourself as an individual, free from comparison and the need for external validation.

Release Self-Judgment

Let go of self-judgment and embrace self-acceptance. Instead of dwelling on perceived flaws or mistakes, focus on your strengths and the progress you have made. Understand that making mistakes is a part of being human, and they provide valuable opportunities for growth and learning. Treat yourself with kindness, compassion, and forgiveness, just as you would treat a dear friend.

Practice Self-Care

Nurture your mind, body, and soul through self-care practices. Dedicate time to activities that bring you peace, joy, and rejuvenation. This can include engaging in hobbies, practicing mindfulness or meditation, taking care of your physical health, or indulging in activities that promote relaxation and well-being. Prioritizing self-care demonstrates your commitment to self-love and reinforces your worthiness of care and attention.

Cultivate Positive Self-Talk

Become aware of your internal dialogue and transform it into a positive and supportive voice. Replace self-criticism and negative self-talk with affirmations and encouraging statements. Remind yourself of your capabilities, strengths, and the progress you have made. Believe in your abilities and value your unique qualities. Over time, positive self-talk will become a natural and empowering habit.

Set Healthy Boundaries

Establishing healthy boundaries is essential for self-acceptance and self-love. Respect your own needs and set clear limits in relationships and commitments. Learn to say no when needed and communicate your boundaries effectively. By honoring your boundaries, you create a space that promotes self-respect and self-care, allowing you to nurture a deeper sense of self-acceptance.

Surround Yourself with Supportive Relationships

Cultivate relationships that celebrate your strengths, encourage your growth, and provide a safe space for vulnerability. Seek out friends, mentors, or support groups that inspire you and share your journey towards self-acceptance and self-love. By surrounding yourself with positive influences, you can reinforce your own belief in your worth and value.

Tips for Embracing Your Physical Self

It's only when you come to terms with and embrace your physical self that you'll realize you're capable of enjoying all the experiences you've been denying yourself. Stop waiting to have fun until you achieve some ideal physical form. Even though altering your self-perception isn't a walk in the park, it is entirely doable. Here are a few easy steps you can take today toward greater self-acceptance in regard to your physical appearance.

1. Go With Acceptance

In spite of how simple or repetitious it may sound, it is vital that you make the decision to accept whatever comes your way. Being able to make a decision is a very effective action. It gives us the freedom to define who we are and what we're willing to accept as part of our lives, as well as the boundaries between the two. Because of the way your mind works right now, you are probably thinking of ways to bully yourself. You have to make a conscious decision to accept and perhaps even love your current body.

In addition, this decision indicates that you are making an effort to mend your strained ties to your physical form. You've decided to stop being your own worst critic and stop treating yourself badly. Make sure you give yourself some praise for making the decision to accept yourself. It's important to remember that the majority of the mental labor involved in shifting our ideas lies in the decision to do so. You've come a long way to get to this point, and that accomplishment alone is worthy of praise.

The transition from body hatred to body love may feel like too great of a leap to make through the use of affirmations alone. If you're finding it challenging or unrealistic to focus on appreciating your body right now, consider shifting your attention to acceptance. Prioritize accepting your body as it is now rather than loving it. Different from body positivity, this is a sort of body neutrality.

If you frequently criticize your arms in your head, that's a good time to put this into practice. You might be thinking something like, "My arms are so awful and flabby." These are certainly extremely pessimistic thoughts, and by experiencing them we associate a powerful emotional state with our otherwise neutral physique. It would be a positive affirmation of one's body to say, "I love my arms." Some people might find this to be unreal, though.

When you practice body neutrality, you tell yourself things like, "These are my natural hands on my natural body. They are what they are." These are apathetic contemplations with no underlying feeling. In a culture where people often express their feelings through their appearance, it can be extremely freeing to adopt a body-neutral stance.

2. Don't Compare

Have you ever come across the proverb that states, "Comparison is the thief of joy?" Focusing on what you don't have, as you would if you compare yourself to others, can only make you feel worse. Say you encountered someone you believed had a perfect figure and immediately started thinking, "I wish I had that shape."

You are putting out a vibration of lack by dwelling on what you don't have, and this will attract additional experiences of lack unless you change your attention. Instead, you might consciously decide to focus on gratitude throughout this time. If you find yourself thinking negatively about your body after seeing a certain woman, consider shifting your focus to something you're thankful for instead.

3. Avoid Body-Shaming Other Women

The acceptance and love of your own body is a prerequisite for the acceptance and love of other women's bodies. Judging another woman based on her appearance reinforces your belief that your own value is determined solely by your physical appearance. You're telling yourself over and over that a person's physical form is fair game for criticism and judgment. In the same way that learning to love ourselves opens the door to naturally loving others, learning to love and accept other people's bodies does the same for us.

A lot of the time, when we find fault with another person, it's because we find fault with that same quality in ourselves. It's a sign that we have bad feelings about our own bodies if we have a negative reaction to someone else's body because of their physique.

Instead of passing quick judgment on someone based on how they seem, try paying them a compliment. Though it would benefit both of you, you need not tell them. You don't have to verbalize the compliment if you don't feel confident doing so. Changing your perspective from criticism to acceptance of others can help you do the same for yourself.

4. Affirm Self-Love Realistically

We may alter our thought processes and even our core beliefs by using affirmations. They provide a direct route for altering our mental processes at both the conscious and subconscious levels. The words we use to describe ourselves have a profound impact on our experiences. This is due to the fact that we build our lives out of the sum of the decisions we make, starting with our thoughts.

Affirmations help us change our critical inner monologue and set off a chain reaction of upbeat thoughts and feelings. To help you remember to love your body each day, write out an affirmation and read it aloud whenever you need a reminder. What matters most about affirmations are not so much the words themselves as the emotions they evoke in you. This is why it's crucial that the affirmations you make come from a place of genuineness. As an added bonus, you should believe in what you're saying.

To say, "I adore my body," when you feel nothing but hatred for your physical form, is an unconvincing lie. This is in direct opposition to how you feel right now, so it may seem impossible to achieve. Make up affirmations you can wholeheartedly believe in instead. Here are some examples of affirmations that get you thinking:

- What I look like is the least intriguing aspect of who I am.

- I will do my best to learn to love and accept my body just as it is.

- My physical form is worthy of my admiration.

These affirmations can be read aloud either before you get out of bed or before you turn in for the night. You may set them as alarms on your phone and have them appear at convenient times throughout the day.

5. Be Grateful for Your Body

In today's image-obsessed culture, it's easy to lose sight of the fact that your physical body serves a purpose beyond vanity. There are innumerable functions in your body, the majority of which are essential to maintaining your health and safety. Regularly remind yourself to appreciate your body for more than just how it looks.

Express gratitude to your physical self for safeguarding your internal organs, facilitating your enjoyment of tasty treats, and receiving the embrace of those you hold dear. The human body is capable of amazing feats that we sometimes take for granted. Practicing gratitude can help you appreciate it more fully.

6. Fight Back Against Fat Prejudice

How do you feel when you hear the word "fat?" Can you think of anything that might make someone feel bad about using it? Is the thought of becoming overweight terrifying, or does it make you feel hateful? The dread or dislike of being overweight is known as fatphobia. The culture condemns obesity as a moral failing.

It may help to question what exactly is wrong with being overweight and to push back against this notion. Would that make them bad people? Does that make a person unworthy? Naturally, it doesn't work like that. Both extreme obesity and stress are known to negatively impact health. In contrast to being overweight, those who are stressed out rarely come under criticism.

In contrast, many people who aren't obviously overweight also experience the same health problems, but they aren't stigmatized in the same manner as those who are visibly overweight. It's the price we pay for being part of a fat-shamed culture. Do some introspection on how you feel about your weight and what it means to you. If you suspect that you harbor fat prejudice, rather than condemning yourself, try learning more about the origins of your beliefs and attitudes. Countering these ideas can lead to a more positive perspective of your physical self.

7. Get Rid of the Weight Scale

Cover up or get rid of your scale. Daily weigh-ins on the scale may make or break the day for many women who have self-esteem issues related to their bodies. There is a continuous ebb and flow to our weight. Fat, muscle, water, and bone density are all factors in one's overall weight. On the scale, two women who appear to have very distinct body types may actually have identical weights. Due to their dissimilar physical make-up, that's the case.

The scale's inability to move after a week of careful food intake and regular exercise can be devastating. The fact is it has nothing to do with your weight. The way you feel is what matters. How well you treat yourself is the key. Get rid of the scale if you find yourself worrying about it or feeling like it has too much power over your life. Nothing good comes from obsessing like this, and it doesn't provide any insight into your true health status. You should pay more attention to how you feel and how well you've been behaving yourself.

8. Reframe Your Approach to Exercise

You may improve your connection with self-care and exercise by changing your mindset about the former. It's common to feel the need to justify a subsequent workout by claiming that you ate something you came to regret afterward. As a result, a negative association is formed between punishment and physical activity.

Instead of viewing exercise as a chore, try viewing it as an opportunity for physical expression and happiness. There are many other benefits to going out besides physical transformation. Its goals are to maintain our physical well-being, ease our minds, and make us happy.

Many activities might count as an exercise toward the goal of maintaining a healthy body and lifestyle. If you hate running and it brings you nothing but misery, there's no use in doing it. Instead, you may enroll in a dance class if that's something that interests you. Working out doesn't have to seem like a punishment or a burden. Determine a physical activity that you look forward to doing and that you can enjoy thoroughly.

Chapter 2:

Embracing Sensuality and Feminine Power

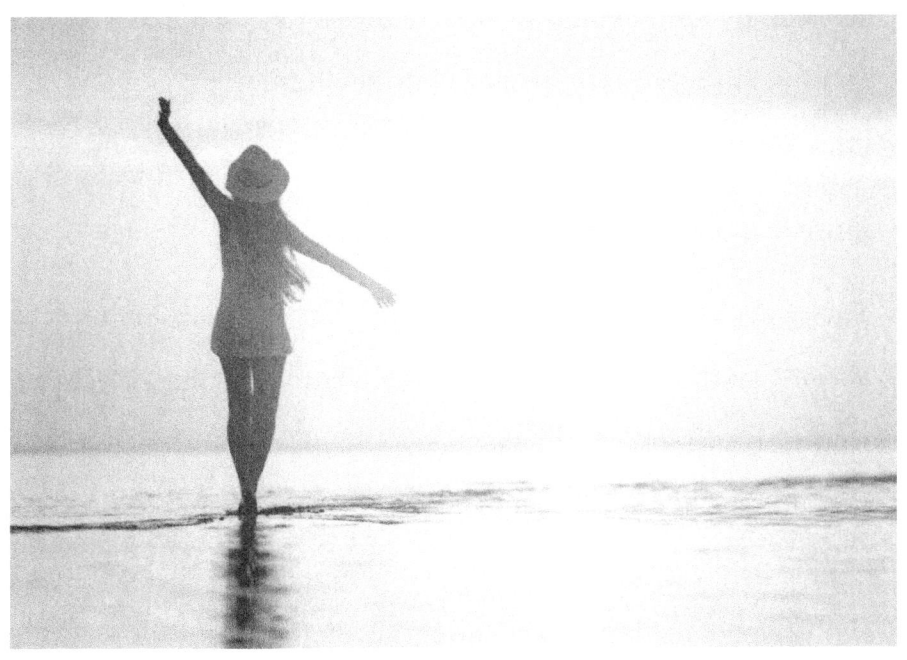

Get to Know the Archetype of the Femme Fatale

The femme fatale archetype has long captivated audiences with her irresistible charm, alluring beauty, and dangerous nature. Originating in ancient mythology and gaining prominence in literature, film, and popular culture, the femme fatale has become an iconic figure that embodies the dark feminine energy. In this exploration, we delve into the depths of this enigmatic archetype, examining her origins, characteristics, and cultural significance. From her historical roots to her modern-day representations, the femme fatale continues to intrigue and provoke discussions about femininity, power, and agency. By understanding the allure and complexity of the femme fatale, we gain insights into the human psyche and the intricate dynamics between desire, danger, and deception.

Historical and Literary Origins

The archetype of the femme fatale can be tracked back to ancient mythology and folklore in many places throughout the world. In Greek mythology, figures like Circe and Medea exemplified the allure and treachery associated with this archetype. Their seductive powers and cunning manipulation showcased the dangerous potential of feminine allure. This theme continued in medieval literature, with characters like Morgan le Fay and Lady Macbeth embodying elements of the femme fatale.

However, it was in the late 19th and early 20th centuries that the femme fatale archetype gained significant prominence in literature. The works of French authors like Charles Baudelaire and Gustave Flaubert explored the concept of the femme fatale, presenting her as a captivating, alluring figure who entices men into ruin and self-destruction. Baudelaire's poem "La Beauté" and Flaubert's novel "Madame Bovary" are prime examples of the portrayal of the femme fatale during this era.

Evolution and Transformation

As the femme fatale archetype made its way into the 20th century, it underwent a transformation that reflected changing social and cultural dynamics. In film noir of the 1940s and 1950s, the femme fatale became a central figure, often portrayed as a dangerous and seductive woman who lures men into criminal activities or leads them to their demise. Iconic characters like Phyllis Dietrichson in "Double Indemnity" and Kathie Moffat in "Out of the Past" illustrate the cunning and manipulative nature of the femme fatale in this era.

In more contemporary times, the femme fatale archetype has continued to evolve, challenging traditional notions of femininity and power. Characters like Catherine Tramell in "Basic Instinct" and Lisbeth Salander in "The Girl with the Dragon Tattoo" embody a modern take on the femme fatale, combining intelligence, sexuality, and assertiveness. These portrayals blur the lines between victim and perpetrator, raising questions about agency and moral ambiguity.

The Seductive Enigma

The allure of the femme fatale lies in her seductive enigma, which combines beauty, intelligence, and a hint of danger. She is often depicted as an empowered figure who uses her sexuality and charm as a means of manipulation and control. The femme fatale's ability to captivate and ensnare her male counterparts stems from the power dynamics inherent in these relationships. Her seductive nature becomes a tool for subverting societal expectations and challenging traditional gender roles.

The duality of the femme fatale is a key aspect of her allure. On one hand, she embodies vulnerability, often presenting herself as a damsel in distress. This vulnerability, however, is a façade that masks her true intentions and cunning nature. By playing on the desires and weaknesses of those around

her, the femme fatale exerts her power and control over them, leaving them spellbound and at her mercy.

The complexity of the femme fatale archetype lies in her ability to subvert societal norms and expectations of femininity. She defies traditional roles of passivity and innocence assigned to women, instead embracing her sexuality and using it as a weapon. This defiance challenges the established power dynamics and brings to the forefront questions about agency and autonomy.

It is important to note that the femme fatale archetype is not inherently negative or villainous. While she often engages in morally questionable actions, her agency and independence can be seen as a rebellion against restrictive societal norms. By embracing her own desires and ambitions, she breaks free from the constraints placed upon women, albeit in unconventional and sometimes destructive ways.

The femme fatale archetype has also been subjected to misconceptions and stereotypes. She is sometimes reduced to a one-dimensional seductress or a femme fatale with no agency of her own, merely a plot device for the male protagonist's journey. However, a closer examination reveals the multidimensionality of the femme fatale. She is a complex character with her own desires, motivations, and vulnerabilities, capable of exerting power and influencing the narrative.

In popular culture, the femme fatale continues to thrive, taking on new forms and narratives. Whether in literature, film, or television, she remains a captivating figure who challenges and intrigues audiences. The fascination with the dark feminine energy she embodies speaks to our collective fascination with the allure of danger and the blurred boundaries between good and evil.

How to Be Sensual and How to Free Yourself from Sexual Bias, You Can Say Goodbye to Shame

As a woman, exploring and embracing your sensuality can be a powerful and liberating experience. It allows you to connect with your own desires, pleasure, and body in a way that is authentic and fulfilling. At the same time, freeing yourself from sexual bias and shedding any feelings of shame can empower you to embrace your sexuality without societal constraints.

Embracing Sensuality

- Self-Awareness: Start by cultivating self-awareness and understanding your own desires and boundaries. Take the time to explore your body, discover what feels pleasurable, and learn about your erogenous zones. This self-discovery can be done through self-pleasure, reading educational resources, or even seeking guidance from a sex-positive therapist.

- Body Positivity: Develop a positive body image by appreciating and accepting your body as it is. Remember that beauty comes in all shapes, sizes, and forms. Engage in activities that make you feel good about yourself, such as exercise, wearing clothes that make you feel confident, and practicing self-care.
- Mind-Body Connection: Cultivate a strong mind-body connection by being present and mindful during intimate moments. Focus on the sensations and pleasure you experience, allowing yourself to fully engage in the moment. This can enhance your overall sensual experience and help you feel more connected to your own body.
- Communication: Open and honest communication is key in any intimate relationship. Express your desires, boundaries, and preferences with your partner(s). Effective communication ensures that you both understand and respect each other's needs, creating an environment where you can freely explore your sensuality without judgment.

Freeing Yourself from Sexual Bias

- Education: Educate yourself about gender biases, stereotypes, and societal expectations surrounding women's sexuality. Read books, articles, and blogs written by feminists, sex educators, and researchers who challenge traditional views on women's sexuality. This knowledge will help you recognize and dismantle any internalized biases you may have.
- Self-Acceptance: Embrace your sexual desires, preferences, and fantasies without judgment. Understand that your desires are valid and unique to you. Emphasize consent, pleasure, and agency in your sexual encounters, and reject any beliefs that shame or suppress your desires.
- Challenging Societal Norms: Challenge societal norms that perpetuate sexual biases by engaging in conversations, sharing your experiences, and promoting healthy and consensual relationships. Encourage open dialogue about women's sexual liberation and challenge double standards that exist in society.

- Surround Yourself with Supportive Individuals: Surround yourself with individuals who support and uplift you. Seek out communities, online or offline, that celebrate diverse sexual experiences and foster an environment of acceptance and understanding. Having a support system can help you navigate any challenges you may face along your journey towards sexual freedom.

Unleash the Power of Emotional Intelligence and Enhance Intuition

In a rapidly changing world, where technological advancements have become the norm, emotional intelligence and intuition continue to be invaluable assets for personal and professional growth. As a woman, developing and harnessing these skills can empower you to navigate various challenges, make better decisions, build stronger relationships, and lead with authenticity.

Understanding Emotional Intelligence

Emotional intelligence (EI) pertains to our ability to identify, comprehend, and effectively handle both our own emotions and the emotions of others. It encompasses self-awareness, self-regulation, empathy, and social skills. Recognizing the importance of emotional intelligence, renowned psychologist Daniel Goleman categorized its components into five domains:

1. Self-awareness: Cultivating self-awareness involves understanding your emotions, strengths, weaknesses, values, and goals. Engage in self-reflection, practice mindfulness, and seek feedback from trusted individuals to deepen your self-awareness.

2. Self-regulation: Develop the ability to manage your emotions, impulses, and behaviors in a constructive manner. This involves practicing emotional resilience, regulating stress, and cultivating healthy coping mechanisms.

3. Motivation: Enhance your motivation by aligning your goals with your values and passions. Set meaningful objectives, celebrate milestones, and cultivate a growth mindset to fuel your drive.

4. Empathy: Empathy entails understanding and sharing the feelings of others. Strengthen this skill by actively listening, showing genuine interest, and practicing perspective-taking. Recognize the power of empathy in building meaningful connections.

5. Social skills: Effective social skills enable you to navigate relationships, communicate assertively, resolve conflicts, and collaborate. Develop your interpersonal skills through active communication, conflict resolution training, and networking opportunities.

The Power of Intuition

Intuition is an innate, gut-feeling or instinctive knowing that guides our decisions and actions. Although often overlooked or dismissed as irrational, intuition plays a crucial role in decision-making and problem-solving. It taps into our unconscious knowledge and experiences, allowing us to make quick judgments in complex situations. As a woman, embracing and enhancing your intuition can be a valuable asset in various aspects of life.

1. Trusting your instincts: Start by acknowledging and trusting your intuition. Pay attention to the subtle cues and sensations that arise within you when making decisions. By embracing and trusting your instincts, you can tap into a wellspring of wisdom.

2. Enhancing self-awareness: Deepening your self-awareness can enhance your intuitive abilities. Regularly

engage in self-reflection, meditation, and mindfulness practices to attune yourself to your inner voice. Journaling can also be a valuable tool to identify patterns and themes in your thoughts and feelings.

3. Listening to your body: Our bodies often provide signals and sensations that inform our intuition. Pay attention to physical cues, such as a feeling of discomfort or ease, a quickening heartbeat, or a sense of calmness. By tuning into your body's wisdom, you can make more aligned choices.

4. Balancing logic and intuition: While logic and rationality have their place, learning to balance them with intuition can lead to more holistic decision-making. Intuition can offer insights that may not be immediately apparent through logical analysis. Allow yourself to explore unconventional or non-linear approaches to problem-solving.

5. Practicing discernment: As you develop your intuition, it is important to cultivate discernment. Not every intuitive insight is accurate or applicable in every situation. Seek

validation, gather additional information, and consider different perspectives to make informed choices.

Enhancing Emotional Intelligence and Intuition in Practice

Emotional Intelligence and Relationships

- Active listening: Practice active listening by fully engaging with others, maintaining eye contact, and providing verbal and nonverbal cues to show understanding and empathy.
- Empathetic responses: Develop the ability to understand and validate others' emotions by responding with empathy and compassion. Acknowledge their feelings and provide support when needed.
- Conflict resolution: Utilize emotional intelligence skills to navigate conflicts effectively. Stay calm, listen to all parties involved, seek common ground, and find solutions that consider everyone's needs and emotions.
- Building rapport: Use your emotional intelligence to build meaningful connections and rapport with others. Be genuine, show interest in their perspectives, and engage in open and honest communication.

Emotional Intelligence and Self-Management

- Stress management: Develop strategies to cope with stress and prevent it from overwhelming you. This may include practicing mindfulness, engaging in relaxation techniques, and maintaining a healthy work-life balance.
- Emotional resilience: Cultivate resilience by recognizing and managing negative emotions effectively. Build a support network, engage in self-care activities, and practice reframing negative situations to maintain a positive outlook.
- Self-motivation: Set clear goals and establish a sense of purpose to stay motivated. Break bigger goals into smaller, achievable tasks, and celebrate your progress along the way. d. Time management: Utilize emotional intelligence to prioritize tasks, delegate when necessary, and set boundaries to ensure a healthy work-life balance. Recognize when to say no and when to ask for help.

Enhancing Intuition

- Cultivating stillness: Set aside time for silence and solitude to quiet the mind and connect with your inner voice. This could include activities such as journaling, meditation, or spending time in nature.

- Trusting your instincts: Practice making small decisions based on your intuition and observe the outcomes. Over time, this will build confidence in your intuitive abilities and allow you to trust them in more significant choices.
- Seeking diverse experiences: Expose yourself to a variety of experiences and perspectives to broaden your intuitive insights. Engage in activities outside your comfort zone and embrace new challenges.
- Developing mindfulness: Practice being fully present in each moment, observing your thoughts and feelings without judgment. Mindfulness enhances your awareness and attunement to your intuitive signals.
- Reflecting on past experiences: Look back on situations where you relied on intuition and assess the accuracy of your intuitive judgments. Learn from these experiences and use them to refine your intuition moving forward.

Chapter 3:

Set Your Own Rules: Find Out How to Defy Expectations and Create Your Own Path

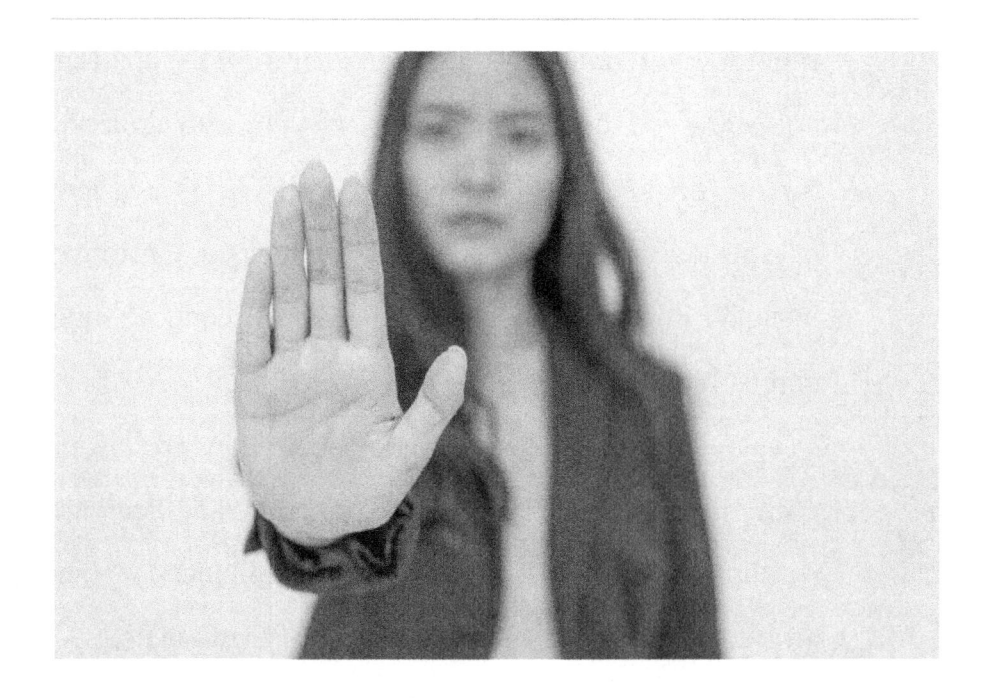

Free Yourself from Gender Roles and Stereotypes

Gender roles and stereotypes have long constrained women, dictating societal expectations and limiting their potential. Nevertheless, in recent yrs, there has been a rising movement towards challenging these norms and empowering women to break free from the confines of gender roles. This section aims to explore the significance of freeing oneself from gender roles and stereotypes as a woman, emphasizing the importance of embracing authenticity and equality. By examining the impact of gender roles on women's lives, understanding the root causes of stereotypes, and discussing strategies to overcome them, we can foster a more inclusive and equitable society for women to thrive.

The Impact of Gender Roles

Gender roles encompass a set of societal expectations and behaviors assigned to individuals based on their gender. Historically, women have been assigned roles as caregivers, homemakers, and supporters, while men have been expected to be providers, leaders, and decision-makers. These roles have perpetuated inequality by limiting women's opportunities for education, career advancement, and leadership positions. The impact of gender roles includes:

1. Limited opportunities: Gender roles often restrict women's access to education, career choices, and economic independence. This contributes to the gender pay gap and the underrepresentation of women in certain fields.

2. Reinforcement of stereotypes: Gender roles reinforce stereotypes about femininity, masculinity, and the idea that certain traits or behaviors are appropriate or expected based on one's gender. This perpetuates harmful stereotypes that limit individuality and self-expression.

3. Psychological effects: The pressure to conform to gender roles can lead to psychological distress, low self-esteem, and a sense of dissatisfaction. Women may feel compelled to prioritize others' needs over their own and suppress their aspirations and ambitions.

Understanding Stereotypes

Stereotypes are oversimplified generalizations or beliefs about a particular group, often based on preconceived notions or biases. Gender stereotypes create a rigid framework that defines how women should look, behave, and fulfill their roles in society. Understanding the origins and impacts of stereotypes is crucial for challenging and dismantling them. Key points to consider include:

1. Cultural and historical influences: Gender stereotypes are deeply rooted in cultural and historical contexts.

They are perpetuated through media, literature, and socialization processes, shaping societal expectations of gender roles.

2. Intersectionality: Gender stereotypes intersect with other social identities, such as race, class, and sexuality. This intersectionality compounds the challenges faced by women who do not conform to traditional gender roles, as they may face multiple forms of discrimination and marginalization.

3. Negative consequences: Stereotypes limit women's autonomy, restrict their choices, and undermine their abilities and achievements. They contribute to gender-based violence, body shaming, and the objectification of women.

Strategies for Overcoming Gender Roles and Stereotypes

As a woman, you have the power to challenge and overcome the limitations of gender roles and stereotypes. By defying societal expectations and embracing your authentic self, you can pave the way for personal growth, empowerment, and contribute to creating a more inclusive society. In this section, we will explore in detail various strategies to overcome gender roles and stereotypes. Through education, self-reflection, empowerment, and activism, you can redefine your identity, break free from societal constraints, and live a life aligned with your true aspirations and values.

Education and Awareness

Education and awareness are crucial in dismantling gender roles and stereotypes. By educating yourself and others about gender equality, feminism, and the experiences of women, you can challenge existing norms and promote change. Here are some strategies:

1. Educate yourself: Take the initiative to learn about the history of women's rights movements, feminist theories, and the impact of gender roles and stereotypes. By understanding the larger context, you can gain insights and knowledge to articulate your perspectives effectively.

2. Share knowledge: Engage in conversations about gender equality and challenge stereotypes in your personal and professional circles. Share information, articles, books, and documentaries that shed light on the experiences

and achievements of women. Encourage open discussions to foster understanding and awareness.

3. Promote inclusive education: Advocate for inclusive education that challenges traditional gender roles and provides equal opportunities for all. Support initiatives that encourage girls and women to pursue science, technology, engineering, and mathematics (STEM) fields, conventionally conquered by men.

4. Mentorship and role models: Seek out mentors and role models who have defied gender roles and stereotypes. Learn from their experiences and seek guidance in navigating challenges. Mentorship programs can provide invaluable support, advice, and encouragement.

Self-Reflection and Empowerment

Self-reflection and empowerment are key aspects of overcoming gender roles and stereotypes. By understanding yourself, embracing your strengths, and asserting your rights, you can break free from societal constraints. Here are some strategies to consider:

1. Challenge internalized beliefs: Reflect on your own beliefs and attitudes about gender roles and stereotypes. Identify any internalized biases or limitations that may be holding you back. Question these beliefs and challenge them by embracing the idea that your worth and potential are not determined by your gender.

2. Embrace your authentic self: Discover who you truly are beyond societal expectations. Embrace your passions, interests, and aspirations, regardless of whether they align with traditional gender roles. Celebrate your unique qualities and assert your right to live a life true to yourself.

3. Build self-confidence: Cultivate self-confidence by recognizing and celebrating your accomplishments, both big and small. Surround yourself with positive affirmations and supportive people who believe in your abilities. Engage in activities that boost your self-esteem, such as practicing self-care, setting and achieving goals, and challenging yourself to step out of your comfort zone.

4. Establish boundaries: Learn to establish clear boundaries and assert yourself when faced with expectations or stereotypes that do not align with your values. Communicate your needs and desires with confidence and respect. By setting boundaries, you protect your autonomy, well-being, and authenticity.

5. Develop assertiveness skills: Practice assertive communication to express your opinions, needs, and boundaries effectively. Use "I" statements to express yourself and assert your rights without diminishing others. Stand up for yourself in situations where you encounter discrimination or unfair treatment.

6. Seek support networks: Surround yourself with like-minded individuals who support and empower you. Seek out communities, organizations, or support groups that promote gender equality and provide a safe space for sharing experiences and seeking advice. Engaging with a supportive network can provide validation, encouragement, and a sense of belonging.

7. Engage in personal development: Invest in your personal growth and development. Attend workshops, seminars,

or training programs that focus on self-empowerment, leadership skills, and overcoming gender stereotypes. Continuously expand your knowledge, skills, and perspectives to enhance your confidence and ability to challenge societal expectations.

Activism and Advocacy

Taking an active role in activism and advocacy is a powerful way to challenge gender roles and stereotypes on a broader scale. By using your voice and platform, you can contribute to the collective effort of achieving gender equality. Here are some strategies to consider:

1. Speak out against gender bias: Challenge gender biases and stereotypes whenever you encounter them. This can be done through engaging in discussions, sharing your experiences, and debunking myths. Advocate for equal opportunities and fair treatment for women in all spheres of life.

2. Support gender-inclusive policies: Stay informed about policies that impact gender equality and advocate for their implementation. This may include advocating for equal pay, family-friendly work policies, and initiatives that address gender-based violence and discrimination.

3. Volunteer and support women-focused organizations: Get involved with organizations that champion women's rights and gender equality. Volunteer your time, skills, or resources to support their initiatives and campaigns. By actively participating in these organizations, you contribute to creating meaningful change.

4. Use social media platforms: Influence social media platforms to raise awareness and challenge gender roles and stereotypes. Share empowering messages, personal stories, and educational content that promote gender equality. Engage in discussions and amplify the voices of other women who are defying expectations.

5. Encourage diverse representation: Advocate for diverse representation in media, politics, and leadership positions. Call for equal opportunities for women from all backgrounds and intersectional identities. Support

and celebrate the achievements of women who break barriers and challenge stereotypes.

6. Mentor and empower others: Pay it forward by mentoring and empowering other women. Share your knowledge, experiences, and insights with those who are navigating similar challenges. By supporting and lifting each other up, we create a stronger and more united front against gender roles and stereotypes.

7. Engage in grassroots movements: Join grassroots movements that fight for gender equality and challenge oppressive systems. Participate in rallies, demonstrations, and campaigns that raise awareness and advocate for change. Your active involvement can help bring attention to the issues and drive collective action.

Find Out Which Are Your Values and Beliefs

Discovering and understanding your values and beliefs is a personal and introspective process. It involves self-reflection, exploration, and critical thinking. Here are some steps you can take to help identify your values and beliefs:

1. **Self-reflection**: Set aside dedicated time to reflect on your thoughts, feelings, and experiences. Consider your past and present, and think about the following questions:

- What is truly important to you in life?
- What principles guide your decision-making process?
- What brings you a sense of fulfillment and purpose?
- What do you stand for and believe in?

2. **Explore your influences:** Consider the people, experiences, and cultural or social environments that have shaped your perspectives. Think about:

- How have your family, friends, and community influenced your values and beliefs?
- Have there been any momentous life events that have impacted your worldview?
- What books, movies, or art have resonated with you and influenced your thinking?
- How has your education or professional background shaped your values?

3. **Engage in critical thinking:** Challenge your assumptions and beliefs by critically analyzing them. Ask yourself:

- Why do I hold these particular beliefs?
- Are there any inconsistencies or conflicts within my values?
- Are my beliefs based on evidence, personal experiences, or societal conditioning?
- Am I open to considering different perspectives and adjusting my beliefs accordingly?

4. **Seek diverse perspectives:** Engage in conversations and seek out diverse viewpoints. This can help you broaden your understanding and challenge your existing beliefs. Consider:

- Participating in discussions with people who have different backgrounds and experiences.
- Reading books or articles from various authors with differing perspectives.
- Actively listening to others and trying to understand their points of view.

5. **Live your values:** Put your beliefs into action. Reflect on whether your behaviors align with your identified values and beliefs. Consider:

- How do your values manifest in your relationships, career, and personal life?
- Do your actions align with your identified beliefs?
- Are there any areas of your life where you can make changes to better live in accordance with your values?

Remember, the process of identifying your values and beliefs is ongoing and may evolve over time. Be patient with yourself and allow room for growth and adaptation. It's also important to note that as a woman, your values and beliefs may be influenced by your gender identity and the unique experiences associated with it.

How to Establish Boundaries and Assert Yourself

Many women are aware of the meaning of the word "boundaries," but they do not understand what the term actually refers to. Typically, we associate boundaries with physical barriers like property lines or figurative "brick walls" that serve to restrict access. However, a boundary is not a set of fixed lines that can be clearly seen by everyone or drawn in the sand. Setting healthy limits and limits for others is an important part of self-care.

Recognizing the Need for Boundaries

To build better boundaries, it is essential for women to first recognize the importance of boundaries and the impact they have on their lives. This section discusses key points related to recognizing the need for boundaries.

1. Self-awareness: Women should develop self-awareness to identify their own emotions, limits, and comfort levels. By paying attention to their feelings and reactions, they can recognize situations where boundaries may be necessary.

2. Respecting personal needs: Women should acknowledge their own needs and prioritize self-care. Understanding that their needs are valid and deserve to be met empowers them to establish boundaries that protect their well-being.

3. Identifying boundary violations: Recognizing instances where others consistently disrespect boundaries or disregard feelings is crucial. Women need to be aware of

such violations to understand the necessity of setting and enforcing boundaries for healthier relationships.

Understanding Different Types of Boundaries

Boundaries come in various forms, each playing a vital role in maintaining healthy relationships and personal well-being. Here are the different types of boundaries that women should be aware of and utilize as needed.

- Physical boundaries: Physical boundaries involve setting limits on touch, personal space, and physical interactions. Women should assert their preferences and communicate their comfort levels clearly and confidently.
- Emotional boundaries: Emotional boundaries protect one's emotions, thoughts, and personal experiences. Women should learn to differentiate between their own emotions and those of others, ensuring they have space to process their feelings without taking on others' emotional burdens.
- Time boundaries: Time boundaries involve managing one's time effectively, prioritizing commitments, and learning to say "no" when necessary. Women should

understand the value of their time and set boundaries around it, ensuring it aligns with their priorities and well-being.

- Intellectual boundaries: Intellectual boundaries encompass respecting and valuing one's thoughts, opinions, and beliefs. Women should assert their right to have their own perspectives while engaging in constructive conversations and respecting the boundaries of others.
- Material boundaries: Material boundaries involve setting limits around personal possessions, finances, and resources. Women should establish guidelines for sharing or lending belongings, avoiding feeling obligated to give beyond their means.

How To Set Boundaries

In today's society, women often face numerous challenges that can impede their personal growth, self-esteem, and overall well-being. The ability to set and maintain boundaries is crucial for women to navigate these challenges effectively. Here's how you can set boundaries effectively and confidently.

1. Understand Your Values and Needs

The first step in setting boundaries is gaining a clear understanding of your values and needs. Take the time to reflect on what is important to you, both in general and within specific relationships or situations. Identify the behaviors, actions, or situations that make you uncomfortable or compromise your well-being. This self-awareness will provide a solid foundation for establishing boundaries aligned with your values.

2. Communicate Clearly and Directly

Effective communication is key when setting boundaries. Clearly and directly express your limits, needs, and expectations to others. Use "I" statements to avoid sounding accusatory or confrontational. For instance, instead of saying, "You always make me feel guilty," try saying, "I feel guilty when..." Be assertive and confident in your communication, expressing your boundaries with respect and without apology.

3. Practice Self-Validation

Setting boundaries often involves going against societal norms or other people's expectations. It is essential to validate your own feelings and needs, even if they differ from others'.

Understand that your boundaries are valid and important, regardless of external opinions or pressures. Trust yourself and your judgment, and remind yourself that it is your right to establish boundaries that support your well-being.

4. Start Small and Gradually

Setting boundaries can feel challenging, especially if you are not accustomed to asserting yourself. Begin by setting smaller boundaries and gradually progress to more significant ones. This approach allows you to build confidence and develop a sense of empowerment in enforcing boundaries. Celebrate each step, no matter how small, and use these victories as motivation to continue setting and maintaining boundaries.

5. Learn to Say No

Saying "no" is a powerful boundary-setting tool. It is okay to decline requests or opportunities that do not align with your values, priorities, or capacity. Remember that saying "no" does not make you selfish or uncaring; it is an act of self-care and self-preservation. Practice saying "no" assertively and without excessive explanations or apologies. Trust that you have the right to prioritize your well-being.

6. Recognize and Address Guilt

Guilt is a common emotion that can arise when setting boundaries, particularly for women who are often socialized to prioritize others' needs above their own. Recognize that guilt is a natural response but understand that your well-being is equally important. Challenge and reframe any guilt-inducing thoughts by reminding yourself that setting boundaries is a necessary act of self-care and self-respect.

7. Seek Support

Setting and maintaining boundaries can be challenging, especially if you encounter resistance or pushback from others. Seek support from family members, trusted friends, or support groups who can provide guidance, encouragement, and validation. Surround yourself with people who respect your boundaries and empower you to prioritize your well-being.

8. Practice Self-Care

Self-care is crucial when it comes to setting boundaries. Engage in activities that nurture your physical, emotional, and mental well-being. Prioritize self-care to replenish your energy and strengthen your ability to establish and maintain boundaries effectively. Remember that self-care is not selfish but a necessary practice for maintaining healthy relationships and overall well-being.

9. Be Firm and Consistent

Setting boundaries requires consistency and firmness. Do not waver in enforcing your boundaries once you have established them. Be consistent in communicating and upholding your limits, even if others attempt to challenge or test them. People may push back or try to guilt you into bending your boundaries, but it's important to stay firm and confident in your decisions. Consistently upholding your boundaries sends a powerful message that they are firm and deserving of respect, leaving no room for negotiation.

10. Practice Self-Reflection

Take the time to assess your boundaries periodically and evaluate if they are still serving your needs. Reflect on any challenges or instances where your boundaries were crossed, and consider how you can adjust or reinforce them moving forward. Self-reflection allows you to adapt and grow in your boundary-setting journey.

11. Set Boundaries in Different Areas of Life

Boundaries are applicable to various aspects of life, including personal relationships, work, and social settings. Identify areas where you need to establish boundaries and tailor them accordingly. This might involve setting limits on your time, emotional availability, or personal space. Recognize that boundaries are flexible and can be adjusted based on different circumstances and relationships.

Chapter 4:

Ignite Self-Confidence: Embrace Your Strengths and Overcome Limitations

Say Goodbye to Self-Doubt and Start Cultivating Inner Confidence

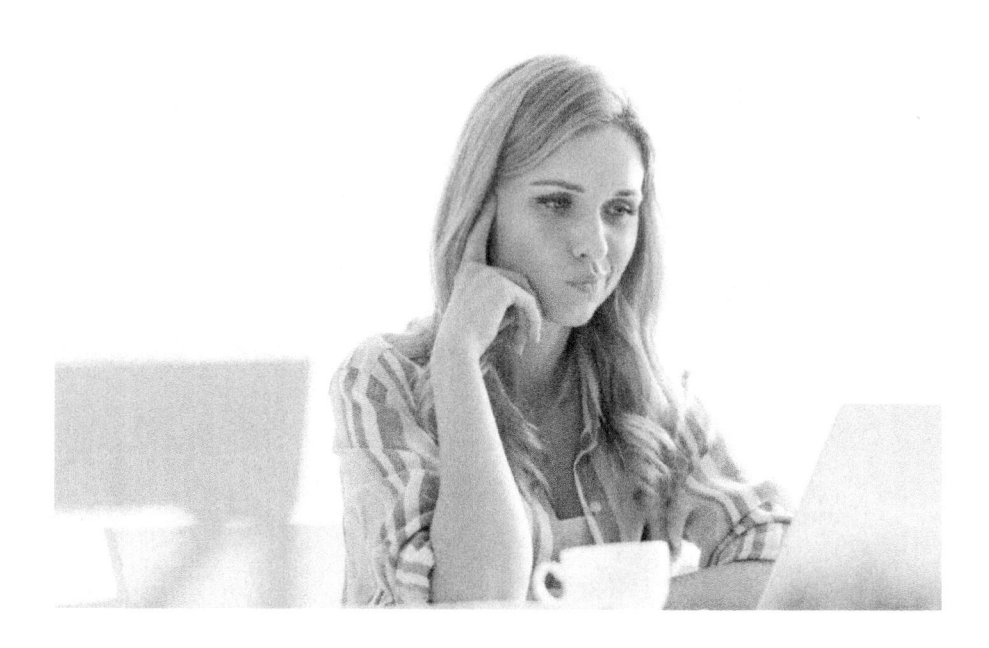

Experiencing self-doubt is all too common, and most of us will have experienced it at one point or another. However, what matters is the way you deal with it, how you cope with it, and what you do with it. It makes all the difference between chronically struggling with self-doubt and allowing it to pass you by. If you keep regularly experiencing self-doubt, you might ask yourself, why does everyone else seem to do well when I'm struggling?

To a certain extent, self-doubt is healthy. Self-doubt enables you to understand when you're not doing something right. With self-doubt, you tend to question and challenge yourself, which prompts internal inquiry. Self-doubt can also bring about humility and increase your understanding of others.

The society we live in values the extraordinary. Therefore, it is common for self-doubt to become a chronic state instead of a fleeting one. When it becomes chronic, you often stand in your own way, and it leads to self-sabotaging thoughts. Even when things are going well for you, you might struggle to see the good. This kind of self-doubt is unhealthy. When you cannot see your good qualities, it becomes difficult to stay motivated. You might believe you will never attain your goals, don't have the talent required, or are unworthy of any position you hold. Any small failure you encounter becomes proof of your perceived sense of unworthiness. Unhealthy self-doubt is like a parasite that consumes you from within while reducing your self-worth, self-esteem, and self-efficacy.

There are certain psychological mechanisms used by self-doubt to perpetuate their unhealthy attitudes toward themselves. For instance, if you're worried that you will not pass an exam, you might be tempted not to study at all. By doing this, you can easily associate the blame of your failure to not studying or the lack of preparation. It is quite an innovative way to shift all the blame away from ourselves and onto an external factor. You can reassure yourself by saying that it was not you who failed, but the situation itself that led to your failure. Had you studied harder, you might have passed. Since you didn't study, you did not pass. This kind of belief is self-sabotaging. Since it stems from the fear of failure, you will always be scared. It is also a reason people tend to procrastinate. If you keep at it for too long, you will eventually reach a situation where you believe you cannot succeed because regardless of what you do, failure is the only potential destination.

The way you talk to yourself repeatedly forms certain dents in your neural pathways. If you keep telling yourself you are incapable of doing something or you are not good enough, these thoughts will become a part of your psyche, and you will believe them to be the truth. This self-fulfilling prophecy is based on the notion that "I cannot." When you convince yourself that you cannot do something, the effort you make will also reduce. If you are going to fail, then what is the point in trying? With less effort, you tend to increase your chances of failing, which in turn reinforces your negative beliefs and ends up creating a rather vicious cycle.

If you don't celebrate your achievements, it is because of a lack of self-kindness. You might be supportive and nurturing towards all those you love, yet you may be critical of yourself. The absence or lack of self-kindness leads to self-doubt. When you are kinder to yourself, it becomes easier to embrace your deficiencies and improve yourself. All those individuals who have a higher level of self-doubt often seek approval from others. They tend to worry more about their failures and negatively evaluate all the situations, which leads to unnecessary self-judgment. It also increases the risk of isolation.

Another factor that is associated with self-doubt is impostor syndrome. It describes an unreasonable feeling of being an impostor where, in fact, all the achievements you attained are accredited to luck instead of your personal abilities and effort. You probably believe that it is only a matter of time before others discover that you are a fraud in disguise. Anxiety and depression are commonly accompanied by impostor syndrome. By giving credit to all your achievements to external factors instead of your own self, you prevent yourself from successfully seeing your self-worth.

Overcoming Self-Doubt
William Shakespeare famously stated that our self-doubts are the same as traitors, and that they force us to miss out on everything beautiful in life since we are so afraid of failing. Self-doubt not only holds you back from acting on opportunities, but it also makes it difficult to start and finish things. The good news is, you can easily overcome self-doubt, provided you make an effort to create change. Self-doubt stems from the internal negative self-talk and wrong beliefs you have formed about yourself. Here are different steps you can use to overcome self-doubt.

Being Real

It is time to be real with yourself. Ask yourself this simple question, "How many times when I feared the worst did it actually become a reality?" Well, if you are honest, then it might not have happened as often as you thought it would. Self-doubts are like the imaginary monsters that kids fear before going to sleep at night. They tend to prevent you from making any changes and keep you well within your comfort zone. If you want to develop and excel in life, you need to step outside your comfort zone.

Take some time and carefully analyze your past. Think about all the instances where things progressed smoothly despite your doubts. Once you realize that not all your self-doubts are based on facts, it becomes easier to let go.

Stop It

Whenever you feel that your internal self-talk becomes negative, tell yourself to stop. You can control your thoughts. Instead of allowing them to spin out of control, you can quickly discourage them. If you feel yourself questioning your own motives, try to talk to the doubtful part in your psyche. You can easily disrupt any patterns of negative self-talk by telling yourself to stop. You can scream at your internal critic to quit being negative. Don't allow your thoughts to control you. Instead, learn to control your thoughts.

Stop Comparing

If you keep comparing yourself to others or to the successes they have attained, it becomes easier to doubt yourself. Since we live in a world where we are surrounded with constant social media posts about others living the perfect life, it becomes tempting to compare oneself with these projections. Instead of comparing yourself to others, compare yourself to yourself. When you spend some time and analyze your life, you will see all the progress you have made. You can be both your biggest opponent and your greatest motivator. The only person you need to outdo is yourself. Think about all the obstacles you have overcome in your life and all the negative circumstances you have successfully navigated. There might have been some instances in your past where you thought it was the end of the world. Well, it wasn't, and the proof is the fact that you are here today! Congratulate yourself on making it this far and keep pushing forward.

Talk to Someone

When you keep all your thoughts to yourself, they often become distorted and exaggerated. It might also reach a situation where they are no longer reasonable. All this is true with self-doubt. To remove yourself from such a situation, it is always a good idea to talk to someone else about it. Once you let go and say these things out loud, you will hear how exaggerated your self-doubt has become. When you talk to someone you trust and love, you might be able to see things from a different perspective.

People Don't Care

A person with extremely high levels of self-doubt often believes that others think about what they say or do. When you start worrying too much about what others think or say, self-doubt tends to get a stronger hold over you. Whenever this happens, remind yourself that people don't really care that much. After all, everyone has their own lives to deal with. Even if they make any negative remarks, it all stops there. Things will not bother you unless you permit them to do so. People have to think about themselves, their jobs, or any other aspect of their lives. Since they have all this to do, they won't have that much time to worry about you. So, forget about what others think. It is not your job to change the way others perceive you. As long as you are true to yourself, you have nothing to worry about.

Journalizing

Maintaining a journal is a very good idea in terms of dealing with self-doubt. Maintain a realistic account of your life. Don't forget to include the positive aspects of your life while writing the negative ones. After all, life isn't always that bad. If you look for it, you will realize that there are many things to appreciate in your life. When you start writing down your doubts and fears, it becomes easier to gain a sense of clarity. All the things you are worried about might not seem that catastrophic once you write them down. Apart from this, it also gives you a better perspective of the issue at hand. Whenever you are facing a challenge, start writing the list of pros and cons of different solutions you can use. This is a rational and logical way to deal with a challenge instead of worrying about failure.

Not Always About You

Regardless of what you might choose to believe, everything isn't always about you. Whenever someone criticizes you, it is easy to start doubting yourself. When someone rejects you on a date, it is difficult not to take it personally. However, what if the things others said were never about you? Perhaps your boss criticized you because he was having a bad day at home. The guy you were on a date with didn't want to go on another date because he was still hung up on his ex. Perhaps he had other commitments to deal with. When you think about all the incidents in your life from the perspective of someone else, you will realize that the world doesn't revolve around you. Instead of readily accepting blame for everything, analyze the situation from the other person's perspective.

Setbacks are Temporary

Nothing in life is permanent. Even if it feels like you're going through an incredibly tough time right now, it will pass. A setback is a temporary situation, and you have the power to overcome it. Keep in mind that you are not a failure because you failed in a specific situation. The true failure is when you refuse to learn from your experiences. Everything that happens in your life happens for a reason. Once you understand the reason, you will be a better version of yourself.

Start following these simple, practical tips, and you will see a change in your internal attitude toward yourself and life.

Paint Your Positive Self-Image and Embrace Body Confidence

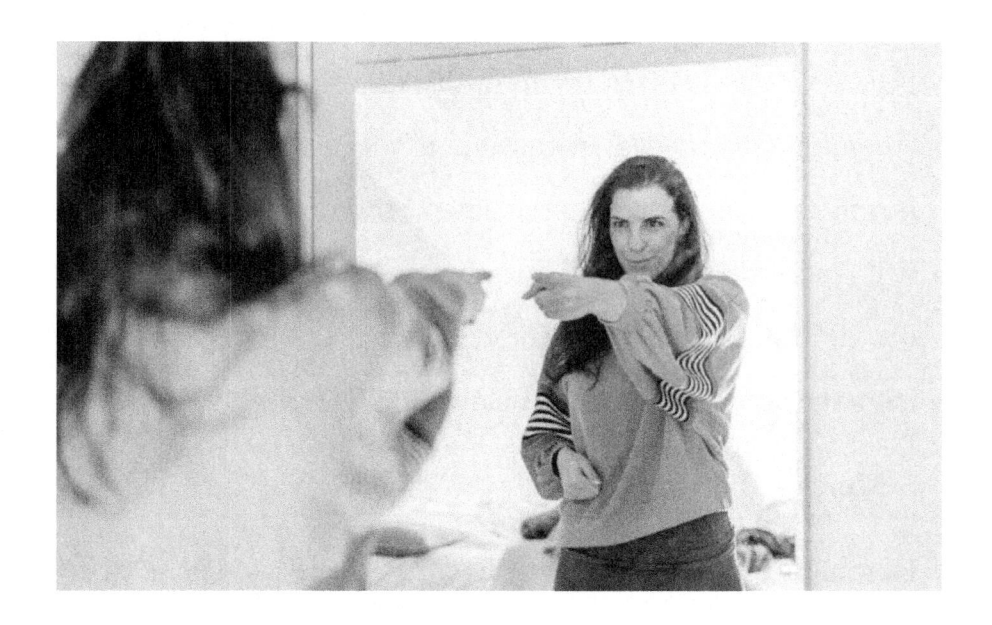

As women, societal pressures and unrealistic beauty standards often challenge our sense of self-worth. However, it is possible to cultivate a positive self-image and embrace body confidence by shifting our mindset and nurturing self-acceptance. Here are the strategies and practices that can help you paint a positive self-image and develop a deep sense of body confidence.

- **Practicing Self-Love**

Practicing self-love is at the core of cultivating a positive self-image and embracing body confidence. It involves treating yourself with kindness, compassion, and acceptance. Begin by acknowledging and appreciating your unique qualities, both physical and non-physical. Focus on your strengths, talents, and achievements, celebrating the aspects that make you who you are.

Make self-care a priority by engaging in practices that nurture your mind, body, and soul. This may involve activities like exercise, meditation, journaling, or pursuing hobbies that bring you joy. Prioritizing self-care communicates a powerful message to yourself that you are worthy of love and care.

Confront negative self-talk and replace it with positive affirmations. Take notice of any negative beliefs or internalized criticisms about your body, and consciously choose to reframe them with statements of self-acceptance and self-love. Surround yourself with positive influences, whether through affirmations, uplifting literature, or supportive social circles.

- **Celebrating Diversity**

Embracing body confidence involves celebrating and honoring the diversity of beauty. Recognize that beauty comes in all shapes, sizes, and forms. Expand your definition of beauty beyond societal norms and challenge the unrealistic standards set by media and advertising.

Seek out diverse representation in the media and follow body-positive influencers who promote self-acceptance and inclusivity. Surround yourself with positive images and messages that reflect a range of body types, ethnicities, ages, and abilities. This exposure helps to normalize and celebrate the diversity of beauty, allowing you to appreciate and embrace your own unique features.

- **Cultivating a Healthy Relationship with Food and Exercise**

Emerging a healthy relationship with food and exercise is crucial in nurturing body confidence. Shift the focus from restrictive diets and punishing exercise routines to nourishing your body and engaging in activities that bring you joy and vitality.

Adopt intuitive eating practices, paying attention to your body's signals of hunger and fullness and allowing yourself to do so will help you lose weight to enjoy a wide variety of foods without guilt or judgment. Focus on nourishing your body with balanced meals that support your overall well-being.

Engage in physical activities that you enjoy and that make you feel good in your body. Move your body in ways that feel joyful and empowering, whether it's dancing, yoga, hiking, or any other form of exercise that resonates with you. The goal is to develop a positive relationship with movement that is based on self-care and self-expression rather than solely on achieving a specific body shape or size.

- **Surrounding Yourself with a Supportive Community**

Building a supportive community is instrumental in fostering body confidence. Surround yourself with friends, family, and mentors who celebrate and uplift you. Seek out communities that promote body positivity, self-acceptance, and self-love.

Engage in open and honest conversations about body image and self-esteem with your loved ones. Share your journey and listen to others' experiences. By creating a safe space for these discussions, you can support one another in embracing body confidence and building positive self-image.

How to Overcome Failures and Learn from Life's Challenges

Life is an unpredictable journey filled with ups and downs, triumphs and failures, and challenges that test our strength and resilience. As a woman, you may encounter unique obstacles and societal pressures that add an extra layer of complexity to your personal and professional life. However, it is essential to remember that failures and challenges are not indicators of your worth or abilities. They are valuable opportunities for growth, self-discovery, and empowerment. In this section, we will explore strategies and mindset shifts that can help you overcome failures and learn from life's challenges, allowing you to thrive and reach your full potential.

- **Cultivate a Growth Mindset**

Developing a growth mindset is a formidable tool for overcoming failures and challenges. Embrace the belief that your abilities and intelligence can expand through dedication and diligent effort. Instead of viewing failures as setbacks or indicators of incompetence, see them as stepping stones toward success. Recognize that failure is an integral part of the learning process and an opportunity for personal growth. By adopting a growth mindset, you empower yourself to persevere, adapt, and learn from every experience.

- **Reframe Failure as Feedback**

Failure is not the end of the road but rather a valuable source of feedback. Shift your perspective and see failures as opportunities to gather valuable insights and learn from your mistakes. Analyze what went wrong, identify areas for improvement, and make adjustments accordingly. Embrace failure as a catalyst for personal growth and development, rather than allowing it to demoralize you. Remember that every successful person has faced failures along the way; it is how they responded and learned from those failures that set them apart.

- **Embrace Self-Compassion**

In the face of failures and challenges, it is crucial to be kind and compassionate toward yourself. Avoid self-blame and negative self-talk, as these only hinder your progress. Treat yourself with the same level of understanding and compassion you would offer a friend. Accept that setbacks are a natural part of life and an opportunity for growth. By practicing self-compassion, you build resilience and foster a positive mindset that enables you to bounce back stronger.

- **Seek Support and Build a Network**

. Facing life's challenges in isolation can be daunting. Foster a network of supportive friends, mentors, and individuals who share your values, as they can offer guidance, encouragement, and valuable perspectives. Look for role models who have triumphed over similar obstacles and gain wisdom from their journeys. Openly communicate your struggles with trusted individuals who can provide valuable advice and unwavering support. Remember, seeking help is a testament to your strength, not a sign of weakness.

- **Take Calculated Risks**

To achieve personal and professional growth, it is essential to venture beyond your comfort zone and embrace risks. Embrace opportunities that test and stretch your limits. While failure is a potential outcome, so is success. Adopt a mindset of ongoing learning and advancement, and be prepared to confront the uncertainty that accompanies risk-taking. Acknowledge and celebrate your courage and resilience, regardless of the outcome, recognizing that each experience contributes to your personal growth journey.

- **Focus on Self-Care**

Amidst life's challenges, it is essential to prioritize self-care. Take care of your physical, emotional, and mental well-being. Participate in activities that bring you joy, help you relax, and recharge your energy. Practice mindfulness, meditation, or other stress-reducing techniques to cultivate emotional resilience. Take time for yourself, nourish your body with healthy habits, and ensure you have a strong support system to lean on during difficult times. When you prioritize self-care, you enhance your ability to cope with failures and challenges effectively.

- **Learn from Successful Women**

Study the stories and experiences of successful women who have overcome failures and challenges. Read biographies, listen to podcasts, or attend events where accomplished women share their journeys. By learning from their wisdom and insights, you gain inspiration and guidance on how to navigate your own obstacles. Identify the strategies they employed to overcome setbacks and implement them in your own life. Remember that their stories serve as proof that failures do not define you but rather provide opportunities for growth and success.

- **Set Realistic Goals and Celebrate Progress**

When faced with failures and challenges, it is crucial to develop goals that are both reasonable and attainable. You can achieve your greater goals by breaking them down into smaller, more doable ones. Rejoice every milestone and accomplishment along the way, as they signify progress and effort. Recognize that setbacks are temporary and do not negate the progress you have made. By focusing on the smaller victories, you build confidence and motivation to keep moving forward, despite the obstacles that may arise.

- **Develop Resilience and Adaptability**

Resilience and adaptability are crucial qualities for overcoming failures and challenges. Life rarely goes according to plan, and unexpected obstacles may arise. Build resilience by learning to bounce back from setbacks, embracing change, and staying open to new possibilities. Develop the ability to adapt your strategies and approaches when faced with unforeseen circumstances. Remember that flexibility and resilience are key ingredients for success in any endeavor.

- **Practice Self-Reflection and Learning**

Take the time to reflect on your failures and challenges. Engage in introspection and ask yourself what lessons you can learn from each experience. Identify patterns or behaviors that may have contributed to the outcome and make a conscious effort to improve upon them. Embrace a growth mindset that views failures as opportunities for self-improvement and learning. Continuously seek knowledge and expand your skill set to enhance your ability to overcome future challenges.

- **Challenge Stereotypes and Bias**

As a woman, you may face additional challenges due to societal stereotypes and biases. Take a stand against these prejudices by challenging them head-on. Advocate for gender equality and diversity in all areas of your life. Surround yourself with individuals who believe in your capabilities and support your aspirations. Remember that your worth and potential are not determined by societal expectations but by your own drive and determination.

- **Stay Persistent and Never Give Up**

Overcoming failures and challenges requires persistence and a refusal to give up. Stay committed to your goals and dreams, even in the face of adversity. Recognize that setbacks are temporary roadblocks and not definitive endpoints. Maintain a positive mindset and believe in your ability to overcome obstacles. Remember that the journey to success is rarely a straight path but rather a series of twists and turns. With persistence, determination, and a growth mindset, you can navigate through any challenges that come your way.

Chapter 5:

Seduction and Magnetism: The Charismatic Presence Way

Find Out Your Unique Charms and Authenticity

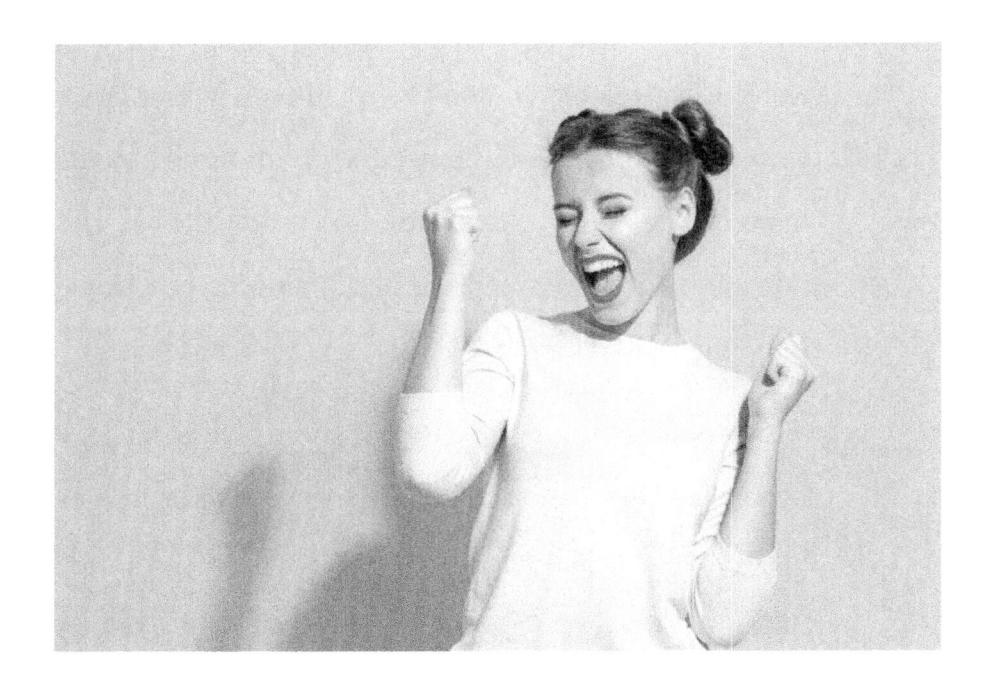

Each woman possesses a distinct set of qualities, experiences, and perspectives that shape her individuality. By embracing and celebrating these characteristics, you can unlock your full potential and radiate your true essence to the world. Let's delve into various aspects that can help you uncover your inner beauty and embrace your authentic self.

1. Embrace your physicality: Your physical appearance is a part of who you are and can be a source of empowerment. Embrace your body, irrespective of societal standards or expectations. Recognize and celebrate the features that make you unique, whether it's the color of your eyes, the texture of your hair, or the shape of your body. Your body is a vessel that carries your spirit, and by accepting and loving it, you exude confidence and charisma.

2. Cultivate self-awareness: Understanding yourself at a deeper level is essential to discovering your unique charms and authenticity. Take time for self-reflection and introspection. Explore your passions, values, strengths, and weaknesses. Consider the experiences that have shaped you and the lessons you've learned along the way. By cultivating self-awareness, you gain clarity about who you are and what truly matters to you,

enabling you to align your actions and choices with your authentic self.

3. Honor your emotions: Emotions are an integral part of the human experience, and as a woman, you possess a unique emotional depth. Allow yourself to feel and express your emotions authentically, whether they are joy, sadness, anger, or vulnerability. Recognize that your emotions are valid and serve as a compass guiding you towards a deeper understanding of yourself. Embracing your emotional landscape fosters a sense of authenticity and enables you to connect with others on a genuine level.

4. Embody self-compassion: Practicing self-compassion is vital in recognizing your unique charms and authenticity. Treat yourself with kindness, love, and forgiveness. Embrace your imperfections and see them as part of your individuality. Celebrate your achievements, no matter how big or small. When you cultivate self-compassion, you create a nurturing space within yourself where you can grow, heal, and flourish authentically.

5. Embrace your passions: Passions are the fuel that ignites your spirit and brings forth your unique talents and gifts. Explore the activities, hobbies, and interests that bring you joy and fulfillment. Whether it's painting, writing, singing, or dancing, engage in activities that light up your soul. By pursuing your passions, you tap into your creative flow, and your unique charms shine through effortlessly.

6. Nurture meaningful relationships: Your connections with others play a significant role in your journey towards authenticity. Cultivate relationships built on trust, respect, and mutual growth. Cherish the connections that celebrate your uniqueness and inspire you to embrace it wholeheartedly. Meaningful relationships provide a mirror that reflects your authentic self and help you discover aspects of your charm that may have remained hidden.

7. Embrace your voice: Your voice is a powerful instrument that expresses your thoughts, beliefs, and values. Embrace the power of your voice and speak your truth authentically. Share your ideas, opinions, and stories

with confidence and conviction. Whether it's through conversations, writing, or public speaking, let your voice be heard. Embracing your voice allows you to contribute to the world in a way that is unique to you and make a positive impact.

8. Practice self-care: Self-care is a vital component of nurturing your unique charms and authenticity. Prioritize activities that rejuvenate and replenish your energy. Engage in self-care practices that resonate with you, whether it's taking a warm bath, practicing yoga, meditating, going for a nature walk, or indulging in a creative outlet. By nurturing yourself, you create the space to reconnect with your authentic self and radiate your unique charms.

9. Embrace your intuition: As a woman, you possess an innate sense of intuition that can guide you towards your authentic path. Trust your inner wisdom and listen to your gut feelings. Be attuned to the subtle whispers of your intuition and allow it to guide your decisions and choices. Embracing your intuition empowers you to

honor your authentic desires and navigate life with a sense of purpose and authenticity.

10. Embody resilience and self-belief: Life is full of challenges and setbacks, but your resilience and self-belief can help you overcome them and stay true to yourself. Believe in your capabilities and trust that you have the strength to navigate any obstacles that come your way. Embrace the lessons learned from difficult experiences, and let them shape you into a stronger, more authentic version of yourself. By embodying resilience and self-belief, you inspire others and radiate your unique charms.

11. Embrace your femininity: Femininity is a beautiful aspect of womanhood and encompasses a wide range of qualities such as grace, compassion, empathy, and nurturing. Embrace and celebrate your femininity in your own unique way. Embody the qualities that feel authentic to you, whether they align with traditional notions of femininity or not. Embracing your femininity allows you to express yourself fully and embrace your unique charms with confidence and pride.

12. Embrace growth and evolution: Discovering your unique charms and authenticity is an ongoing journey that evolves over time. Embrace growth and be open to change. Allow yourself to explore new interests, challenge old beliefs, and embrace the lessons that life presents. Embracing growth and evolution enables you to continuously uncover new layers of your authentic self and expand your unique charms.

Boost Your Communication and Social Skills

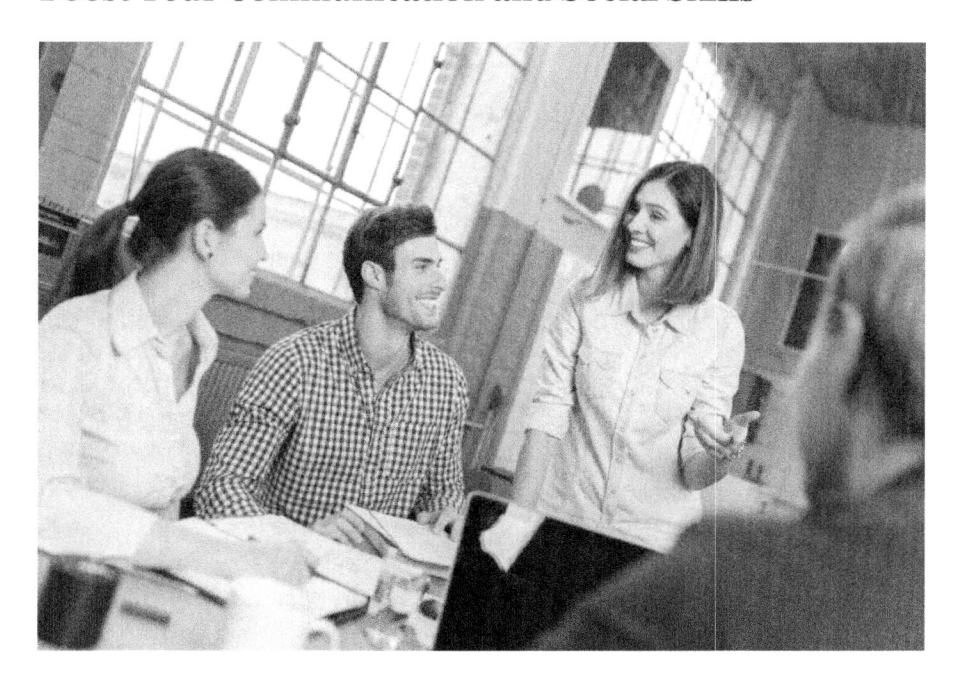

Effective communication and strong social skills are essential for personal and professional success. As a woman, developing these skills can greatly enhance your confidence, relationships, and overall well-being. Whether you're interacting with colleagues, friends, or acquaintances, having the ability to communicate effectively and navigate social situations with ease is crucial. In this guide, we will explore practical strategies to boost your communication and social skills, enabling you to connect more deeply, express yourself confidently, and build stronger connections with others.

Developing Effective Communication Skills

Active Listening:

Active listening is a fundamental aspect of actual communication. It requires completely interacting with the person who is speaking and exhibiting both attention and comprehension in what they are saying. To enhance your active listening skills:

1. Pay attention and focus on the speaker: Eliminate distractions, maintain eye contact, and provide your undivided attention to the person speaking. This

demonstrates respect and shows that you value their input.

2. Demonstrate interest through verbal and non-verbal cues: Nodding, smiling, and using appropriate facial expressions indicate your engagement and encourage the speaker to continue sharing. Verbal cues like "I see," or "Tell me more," show that you're actively listening and interested in their perspective.

3. Ask clarifying questions and provide feedback: Seek clarification when needed to ensure you understand the speaker's message accurately. Paraphrase their key points to show that you've understood and provide constructive feedback to contribute to the conversation.

Assertive Communication

Assertive communication involves expressing your thoughts, needs, and boundaries clearly and respectfully, while considering the rights and needs of others. To boost your assertive communication skills:

1. Express yourself clearly: Use "I" statements to convey your feelings, thoughts, and opinions without blaming or criticizing others. This allows you to express yourself assertively while maintaining respectful communication.

2. Respectful assertiveness: Find the balance between advocating for your needs and considering the perspectives of others. Assertive communication involves standing up for yourself while treating others with empathy and respect.

3. Active listening in assertive communication: Actively listen to others during conversations. Show empathy, seek to understand their viewpoints, and respond thoughtfully, fostering meaningful dialogue and mutual understanding.

Non-Verbal Communication

The significance of nonverbal cues in communication cannot be overstated, often conveying messages beyond words. To enhance your non-verbal communication skills:

1. Body language: Be aware of your posture, gestures, and facial expressions. Maintain an open and relaxed posture, avoid crossing your arms, and use appropriate gestures to support your verbal communication.

2. Eye contact: Maintain appropriate eye contact during conversations to show attentiveness and interest. However, be mindful of cultural differences and individual comfort levels regarding eye contact.

3. Personal space: Respect others' personal space by maintaining an appropriate physical distance during interactions. Be aware of cultural norms and individual preferences regarding personal space boundaries.

Emotional Intelligence

As mentioned earlier, emotional intelligence is defined as an ability to recognize, interpret, and control one's own feelings in a healthy and productive manner, while also displaying empathy towards the emotions of others. To develop your emotional intelligence:

1. Self-awareness: Take time to reflect on your own emotions, triggers, and biases. Understand how your

emotions may influence your communication and strive for self-improvement.

2. Empathy: Practice putting yourself in others' shoes to understand their emotions, perspectives, and experiences. Empathy helps you respond with understanding and compassion, fostering stronger connections.

3. Emotional regulation: Develop strategies to manage your emotions effectively. By recognizing and regulating your emotions, you can respond thoughtfully rather than react impulsively, leading to more constructive communication.

Enhancing Social Skills
Building Rapport

Building rapport involves creating connections and positive relationships with others through genuine engagement and shared experiences. To enhance your rapport-building skills:

1. Find common ground: Look for common interests, hobbies, or experiences to establish a foundation for

conversation. Finding commonalities helps create a sense of connection and fosters meaningful interactions.

2. Demonstrate genuine interest: Show curiosity and actively listen to others. Ask open-ended questions that encourage them to share more about themselves, and actively engage in the conversation by responding thoughtfully.

3. Use open-ended questions: Open-ended questions invite deeper conversation and allow others to express themselves more fully. Instead of closed-ended questions that elicit simple yes/no answers, ask questions that encourage elaboration and provide an opportunity for meaningful dialogue.

Conflict Resolution

Although having disagreements is an inevitable aspect of having interpersonal interactions, having the ability to effectively resolve conflicts is essential to establishing healthy connections. To enhance your conflict resolution skills:

1. Address conflicts constructively: Instead of avoiding or escalating conflicts, address them in a proactive and

constructive manner. Acknowledge the issue and express your concerns or perspectives calmly and respectfully.

2. Active listening and empathy: During conflicts, practice active listening to understand the other person's viewpoint. Show empathy by acknowledging their feelings and demonstrating that you genuinely care about finding a resolution.

3. Finding win-win solutions: Collaborate with the other party to find mutually beneficial solutions. Explore different perspectives, be open to compromise, and focus on finding resolutions that meet the needs of both parties.

Networking and Building Connections

Networking plays a vital role in personal and professional growth. To enhance your networking skills and build stronger connections:

1. Attend events: Actively participate in professional and social events where you can meet new people. This provides opportunities to expand your network and

establish connections with individuals who share similar interests or professional goals.

2. Building relationships: Building relationships takes time and effort. Nurture professional connections by regularly communicating, offering support, and showing genuine interest in others' successes and challenges. Invest in maintaining these relationships through meaningful interactions.

3. Making new connections: Be proactive in making new connections. Introduce yourself, strike up conversations, and show genuine curiosity about others. Take the initiative to initiate follow-ups and explore potential collaborations or friendships.

Developing Social Confidence

Social confidence is key to thriving in social settings and building connections. To develop your social confidence:

1. Overcoming social anxiety: Challenge yourself to step outside your comfort zone gradually. Practice socializing in different settings, and recognize that discomfort is a

natural part of growth. With time and practice, your social confidence will improve.

2. Embracing vulnerability: Be authentic and genuine in your interactions. Share your thoughts, feelings, and experiences openly, allowing others to see the real you. Embracing vulnerability creates opportunities for deeper connections and fosters authenticity.

3. Positive self-talk and a growth mindset: Replace negative self-talk with positive affirmations. Cultivate a growth mindset that views social interactions as opportunities for learning and personal growth. Recognize that mistakes and setbacks are part of the journey and approach each interaction as a chance to improve.

Basics of Magnetic Presence and Attracting Positive Connections

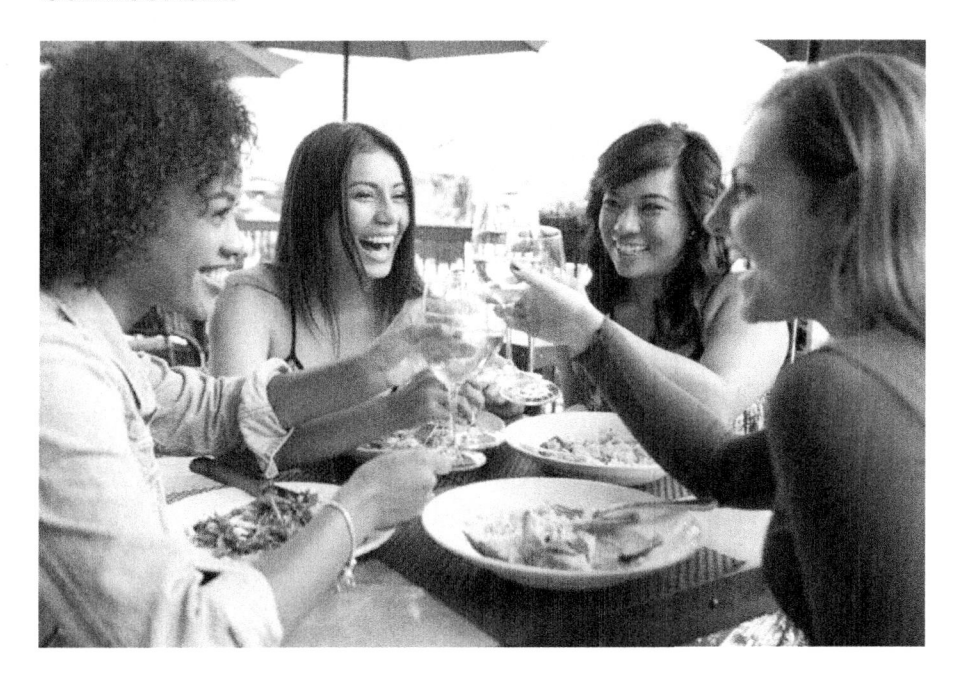

Have you ever heard someone talk and just been in awe of them or watched a video that inspired you to change something about yourself? People who are charismatic have a kind of charm that inspires devotion in those around them. When they talk, everyone listens. They have the ability to make others want to be around them.

These are people who speak with massive confidence and always teach you something or leave you with a different perspective. You can never have a dull moment with such individuals because of how full of life and positive energy they are. They always see the best in situations and other people, bouncing back from setbacks faster than other people. More importantly, they have the capability to encourage others to see the world and life differently, enabling them to be optimistic, too.

Here's the best part: Charisma is a skill; so it's not like you're either born charismatic or you're not—it's a learned behavior! Therefore, you, my girl, can be charismatic. So, what qualities does a charismatic woman have? Here are a few:

- She's self-confident and headstrong.
- She's emotionally intelligent and empathetic.
- She radiates positive energy.
- She's responsible and gets shit done.
- She has a burning desire to always be better and work on her personal growth.
- She has a balance of masculine and feminine energies.

Becoming charismatic will drive people toward you; they will want to learn about your story and become inspired by you. People will start looking up to you, and through your contribution, you will be able to add value to their lives.

As humans, we all have a need for growth and contribution. We aim to live our lives for a purpose that is higher than ourselves and contribute to the betterment of the world. Once we are able to accomplish this, we feel a sense of completeness and delight in that very instant.

7 Easy Ways to Be a Charismatic Woman

Since charisma is a skill you can learn, here are seven quick ways you can start practicing now:

1. Make others feel important

Charismatic women are not self-centered; they are attentive to the experiences of others and take genuine interest in the tales others tell. They ask interesting questions and listen attentively.

When you're talking to someone, make sufficient eye contact and show them that you are interested in what they have to say.

2. Practice speaking expressively

Everyone knows how to speak, but not everyone can speak expressively. In order to be charismatic, speak with your heart, not just your brain. Connect with people on an emotional level while speaking concisely and powerfully. This will make them feel put at ease by your presence.

3. Accentuate your best features

To have charm as a woman does not require you to be the prettiest lady in the room, however about rocking what you have confidently. Shift your focus from trying to hide your perceived flaws toward highlighting what you love most about yourself!

4. Look approachable

Yeah you know that resting bitch face many of us have...? Drop it. Body language says a lot about who you are, so regardless of how kind you may be, if you're always looking like you're about to slap a bitch, people will not approach you.

When someone talks to you, smile at them, turning your knees or face toward them so they feel important around you.

5. Smile regularly

There's something about a smile that is utterly contagious—If a stranger smiles at you, chances are you will probably smile back at them. Try and smile at people as much as possible; they will naturally feel drawn toward you.

6. Tell entertaining stories

Storytelling is a great art, one you may want to perfect. When you're in a crowd of people, tell stories in a way that brings every moment to life so they feel like they are reliving it with you.

7. Be confident

Confidence isn't just about walking into a room with a brave face—it also means having the confidence to be vulnerable and real. People are attracted to authenticity; they feel connected to those who are willing to level with them.

Remember all that you need to be a charismatic woman is already inside you - this book isn't about turning you into someone new; it's about allowing you to tap into your existing potential so that you can unleash your true self.

Chapter 6:

The Art of Seduction: Mastering the Power to Captivate Men

A Journey into the Psychology of Male Attraction

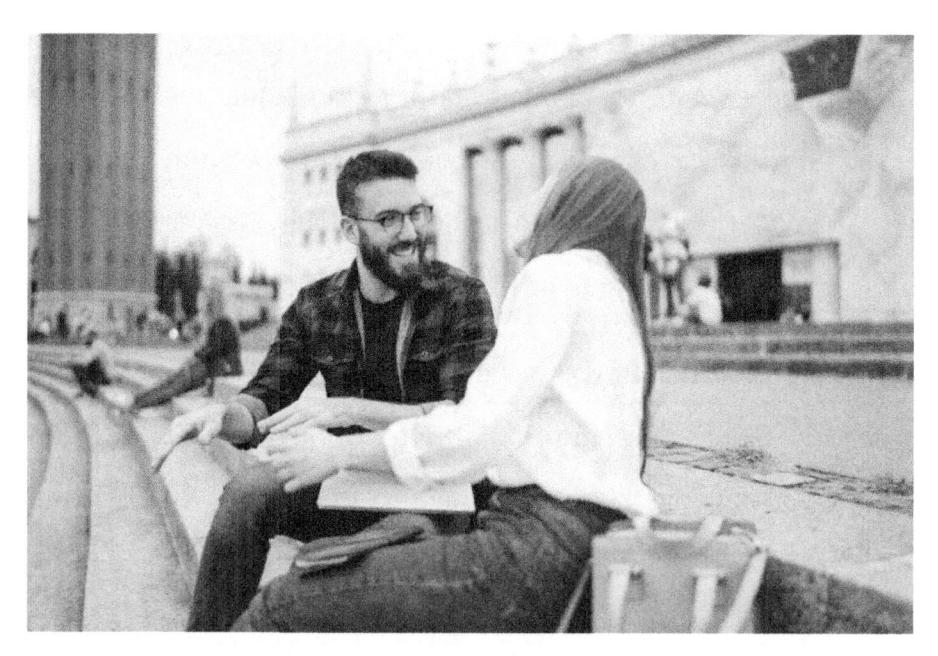

The psychology of attraction has been a subject of fascination for centuries, with numerous theories and studies attempting to unravel its mysteries. While attraction is a complex phenomenon that encompasses various factors, this exploration focuses specifically on the psychology of male attraction. By understanding the psychological processes and mechanisms that drive male attraction, we gain insights into the intricacies of human behavior and the dynamics of romantic relationships. From evolutionary theories to cultural influences, we embark on a journey into the depths of male attraction, exploring its origins, drivers, and implications.

Evolutionary Perspectives on Male Attraction

Evolutionary psychology offers valuable insights into the roots of male attraction. According to evolutionary theories, males are wired to seek certain traits in potential mates that enhance their reproductive success. This perspective suggests that men are attracted to physical cues of fertility and health, such as youthfulness, symmetry, and waist-to-hip ratio. These traits are believed to signal reproductive fitness and the potential to bear healthy offspring. Additionally, evolutionary psychology posits that men are inclined to be attracted to signs of availability and receptivity, such as flirtatious behavior or cues indicating sexual interest.

Cultural Influences on Male Attraction

While evolutionary factors play a significant role in shaping male attraction, cultural influences also come into play. Cultural norms, values, and societal expectations shape perceptions of attractiveness and influence the types of traits and qualities men find desirable in potential partners. Beauty standards, for instance, vary across cultures and can influence men's preferences for certain physical attributes. Media and advertising also play a substantial role in shaping ideals of attractiveness and may impact what men perceive as desirable.

Psychological Factors in Male Attraction

Beyond evolutionary and cultural influences, psychological factors contribute to male attraction. One such factor is interpersonal chemistry or compatibility. Men are often drawn to individuals with whom they share common interests, values, and personalities. The psychological concept of similarity attraction suggests that people are more likely to be attracted to others who are similar to them in various aspects. Shared beliefs, attitudes, and goals can create a sense of connection and understanding, fostering attraction.

Emotional and Intellectual Stimulus in Male Attraction

Attraction goes beyond physical appearance and encompasses emotional and intellectual elements. Emotional attraction is characterized by a deep emotional connection, empathy, and mutual understanding. Men may be drawn to individuals who display warmth, kindness, and emotional intelligence. Intellectual stimulation is another key aspect of attraction. Men are often attracted to individuals who engage them intellectually, challenge their perspectives, and stimulate their curiosity. The ability to engage in meaningful conversations and share intellectual interests can enhance the overall attraction.

The Role of Confidence and Self-assurance

Confidence and self-assurance play a crucial role in male attraction. Men are often attracted to individuals who display confidence, as it signals self-assuredness and assertiveness. Confidence can be perceived as an indicator of social status and the ability to navigate social interactions effectively. Additionally, individuals who are confident in themselves and their abilities tend to exude a positive energy, which can be appealing to others.

The Impact of Personal Experiences and Individual Differences

Personal experiences and individual differences also shape male attraction. Past experiences, such as previous relationships or upbringing, can influence what individuals find attractive. Preferences can be influenced by positive or negative experiences, shaping future preferences and expectations. Individual differences, such as personality traits, attachment styles, and personal values, also contribute to attraction. For example, individuals with a secure attachment style may be more attracted to partners who offer emotional support and security.

The Complex Nature of Attraction

It is important to recognize that attraction is a multifaceted and highly individual experience. While general patterns and tendencies exist within male attraction, it is essential to acknowledge that each individual's preferences and experiences are unique. What one man finds attractive may not necessarily resonate with another. Furthermore, attraction is a dynamic process that can evolve and change over time as individuals grow and develop.

The interplay between biological, psychological, and cultural factors makes the psychology of male attraction a complex and nuanced subject. It is influenced by both conscious and unconscious processes, as well as societal and personal expectations. Understanding the various factors at play can help shed light on the dynamics of romantic relationships and provide insights into human behavior.

It is also crucial to approach the topic of male attraction with sensitivity and respect for the diversity of experiences and preferences. There is no universal standard of attractiveness, and everyone has their own unique set of attractions and desires. It is essential to foster a culture that values individuality and encourages open-mindedness when it comes to exploring and accepting different forms of attraction.

Release Your Seductive Energy and Charisma

Seductive energy and charisma are qualities that can have a profound impact on how we interact with others, build connections, and leave a lasting impression. These traits are not limited to a select few; rather, they can be cultivated and developed by anyone. In this section, we will discuss the art of unleashing your seductive energy and charisma, discovering how to tap into your inner charm and magnetism. By embracing your unique qualities and enhancing your interpersonal skills, you can captivate others and create meaningful connections in various aspects of your life.

Understanding Seductive Energy

Seductive energy is a potent force that emanates from within, captivating others and drawing them towards you. It is a combination of confidence, self-assurance, and authenticity that shines through in your presence and interactions. Seductive energy is not about manipulating or deceiving others; rather, it is about embodying your true self and radiating a magnetic aura that others find irresistible. By understanding and embracing your unique qualities and strengths, you can tap into your seductive energy and exude a captivating charm.

Developing Charismatic Communication

Communication plays a crucial role in expressing your seductive energy and charisma. Developing charismatic communication skills allows you to engage others, create a sense of connection, and leave a lasting impact. Effective communication involves active listening, genuine interest in others, and the ability to express yourself clearly and confidently. It also involves non-verbal cues such as body language, eye contact, and a warm and engaging smile. By practicing and honing your communication skills, you can amplify your seductive energy and make a memorable impression on those around you.

Confidence and Self-Assurance

Confidence and self-assurance are vital ingredients in unleashing your seductive energy and charisma. When you believe in yourself and your abilities, others are naturally drawn to your energy and presence. Cultivate self-confidence by recognizing and appreciating your strengths, setting and achieving realistic goals, and embracing self-care practices that enhance your overall well-being. Embracing a positive mindset and affirming your worth can also contribute to your confidence levels. Remember, confidence is not about being flawless or never experiencing doubt, but rather about accepting yourself fully, including your imperfections, and showing up authentically.

Authenticity and Vulnerability

Authenticity and vulnerability are powerful tools in unlocking your seductive energy and charisma. When you are genuine and vulnerable, you create a space for others to connect with you on a deeper level. Embrace your true self, allowing your unique personality and quirks to shine through. Share your thoughts, emotions, and experiences with others, fostering trust and intimacy. Remember that vulnerability is a strength, as it allows for genuine connections to form. By being authentic and vulnerable, you invite others to do the same and create a genuine bond that goes beyond surface-level interactions.

The Power of Body Language

Body language plays a significant role in expressing your seductive energy and charisma. Your gestures, posture, and facial expressions can convey confidence, openness, and approachability. Maintain an upright posture, with your shoulders back and head held high, to exude confidence and command attention. Use open and inviting gestures, such as maintaining open palms and relaxed arms, to create a welcoming atmosphere. Eye contact is another powerful tool; it shows interest and engagement in conversations. When combined with a warm and genuine smile, eye contact can enhance your seductive energy and create a positive impression on others.

Embracing Your Personal Style

Your personal style is an integral part of unleashing your seductive energy and charisma. It is an expression of your individuality and can greatly impact how you are perceived by others. Discovering and embracing a style that reflects your personality, values, and aspirations allows you to present yourself authentically and confidently.

Experiment with different fashion choices, finding clothing that makes you feel comfortable, empowered, and aligned with your desired image. Pay attention to the colors, patterns, and silhouettes that resonate with you and make you feel your best. Your personal style should be a reflection of who you are and what you want to convey to the world.

Grooming and self-care are also essential aspects of personal style. Taking care of your physical appearance not only enhances your overall attractiveness but also boosts your self-confidence. Find grooming practices that make you feel polished and well put-together, whether it's through skincare, hairstyling, or maintaining a neat and clean appearance.

Developing Emotional Intelligence

Emotional intelligence is a fundamental aspect of seductive energy and charisma. It involves the ability to recognize and understand your own emotions as well as the emotions of others. Cultivating emotional intelligence allows you to navigate social interactions with empathy, authenticity, and sensitivity.

Practice self-awareness by tuning into your emotions and understanding their underlying causes. This awareness enables you to manage your emotions effectively and respond to situations in a composed and emotionally intelligent manner. By regulating your emotions, you create a sense of stability and control that is attractive to others.

Empathy is another crucial component of emotional intelligence. Seek to understand the perspectives and feelings of those around you. Show genuine interest and compassion, and be present in your interactions. This empathetic approach allows you to connect deeply with others and build meaningful relationships.

Continual Growth and Self-Development

Unleashing your seductive energy and charisma is an ongoing journey of growth and self-development. It requires a commitment to personal growth, a willingness to step outside of your comfort zone, and a dedication to learning and improving.

Engage in activities that expand your knowledge, skills, and experiences. Pursue hobbies and interests that ignite your passion and make you feel alive. By constantly challenging yourself and pushing your boundaries, you develop a sense of confidence and charisma that is magnetic to others.

Cultivate a supportive network of individuals who uplift and motivate you. Seek mentors or role models who embody the qualities you admire and can provide guidance along your journey. Engage in positive and empowering conversations that encourage personal growth and self-reflection.

How to Nurture Emotional Connection and Build Intimacy

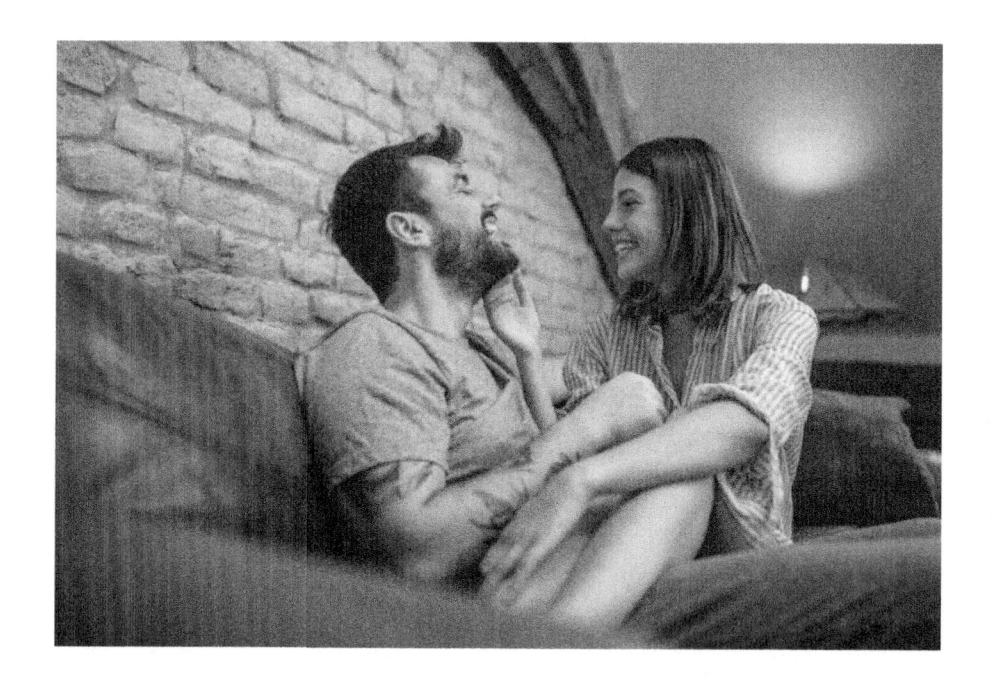

Emotional connection and intimacy are vital components of fulfilling and meaningful relationships. As a woman, you have the power to nurture and strengthen these bonds, fostering deeper connections with your partner. Listed below are practical strategies and insights to help you cultivate emotional connection and build intimacy in your relationships. By embracing vulnerability, effective communication, active listening, trust-building, and prioritizing quality time, you can create a strong foundation for lasting and fulfilling connections.

1. Embrace Vulnerability

Vulnerability is the cornerstone of building emotional connection and intimacy. It involves allowing yourself to be open and authentic, sharing your thoughts, feelings, and fears with your partner. Break down emotional barriers and be willing to express vulnerability, even if it feels uncomfortable at first. When you show your authentic self, it encourages your partner to do the same, fostering trust and deepening the emotional bond between you.

2. Foster Effective Communication

Establishing emotional connection and intimacy relies on effective communication. Foster open and honest communication with your partner, openly expressing your needs, desires, and concerns. Create a secure environment where both of you can share without fear of judgment or criticism. Utilize "I" statements to convey your feelings and actively listen to your partner's viewpoint. Avoid defensiveness and instead strive to understand each other's perspectives. Through effective communication, you can deepen emotional understanding and lay the foundation for a stronger and more connected relationship.

3. Practice Active Listening

Active listening is an indispensable skill for building emotional connection and intimacy. Give your partner your full attention when they are speaking, without interrupting or assuming their thoughts. Show empathy and validate their feelings. Reflect back what they have said to ensure understanding and ask clarifying questions when needed. By practicing active listening, you demonstrate your genuine interest in their thoughts and emotions, fostering a deeper sense of connection.

4. Build Trust

Trust forms the foundation of emotional connection and intimacy. Cultivate trust in your relationship by being reliable and consistent in your actions and words. Keep your promises and commitments, and avoid betraying your partner's trust. Be transparent and honest, even when it is difficult. Trust is built over time through consistent actions that demonstrate your reliability and integrity. By building trust, you create a secure and safe space for emotional connection to flourish.

5. Prioritize Quality Time

Quality time is essential for nurturing emotional connection and intimacy. Create opportunities to spend meaningful time with your partner, free from distractions. Engage in activities that promote connection and bonding, such as having deep conversations, going on dates, or engaging in shared hobbies. Put away electronic devices and be fully present during these moments. Quality time allows you to connect on a deeper level and strengthens your emotional bond.

6. Express Appreciation and Affection

Expressing appreciation and affection is crucial for building emotional connection and intimacy. Show gratitude for your partner's presence in your life and acknowledge their efforts and qualities. Offer compliments and express affection through physical touch, hugs, kisses, and holding hands. Small gestures of love and kindness go a long way in fostering emotional connection and building intimacy.

7. Explore Emotional and Sexual Intimacy

Emotional and sexual intimacy are intertwined and contribute to a strong connection between partners. Engage in open and honest conversations about your desires, boundaries, and fantasies. Explore emotional intimacy by sharing your deepest thoughts, fears, and dreams. Cultivate a safe and non-judgmental environment where both of you can express your needs and desires. Remember that building intimacy takes time, patience, and ongoing communication.

8. Respect and Support Individual Growth

Supporting each other's individual growth is vital for maintaining emotional connection and intimacy. Encourage your partner to pursue their interests, passions, and personal growth. Respect their autonomy and allow them space to explore and develop as an individual. Offer your support, encouragement, and understanding as they navigate their own journey. By respecting and supporting each other's growth, you create a foundation of trust and mutual respect, which strengthens the emotional connection in your relationship.

9. Practice Forgiveness and Letting Go

Forgiveness is an essential element in nurturing emotional connection and intimacy. Holding onto grudges and past resentments creates barriers to deep emotional connection. Learn to forgive and let go of past hurts, understanding that no one is perfect. Communicate openly about the impact of certain actions, but also offer forgiveness and a chance for growth and change. Forgiveness allows both partners to move forward and rebuild emotional trust, fostering deeper intimacy.

10. Prioritize Self-Care

Taking care of your own emotional well-being is crucial for building emotional connection and intimacy in relationships. Engage in self-care practices that promote self-love and self-compassion. Nurture your own emotional needs and ensure you have a healthy balance between personal time and time spent with your partner. When you prioritize your own well-being, you bring a healthier and more vibrant energy to your relationship, enhancing emotional connection and intimacy.

11. Seek Professional Help if Needed

If you find that building emotional connection and intimacy is challenging, consider seeking the guidance of a professional therapist or counselor. They can provide valuable insights, tools, and strategies to help you navigate any underlying issues or barriers that may be hindering emotional connection and intimacy. Seeking professional help is a proactive step towards nurturing a healthier and more fulfilling relationship.

Conclusion: Integrate Your Dark Feminine Energy

By embracing and integrating your dark feminine energy, you have already initiated a powerful process of transformation and growth. As you delve into this journey, you will experience numerous benefits, such as empowerment and authenticity. Empowerment enables you to tap into your inner strength and assertiveness, empowering you to take charge of your life and make choices that align with your true self. Authenticity allows you to live in alignment with your values and beliefs, fostering a genuine and fulfilling existence.

However, it is important to recognize that your journey has only just begun. This path is an ongoing process of self-discovery and self-expression. By exploring the depths of your being and embracing all aspects of yourself, including the dark feminine energy, you unlock a wellspring of creativity, passion, and wisdom.

Embrace the challenges and opportunities that come your way, for they are catalysts for growth and self-realization. Remain open to learning, expanding your horizons, and pushing beyond your comfort zone. Trust in your intuition and inner guidance as you navigate this transformative journey.

Remember, integrating your dark feminine energy is not about conforming to societal expectations, but about embracing your authentic self and embracing the power and beauty within you. Embrace your uniqueness, honor your truth, and let your light shine brightly as you continue to explore, discover, and express your true essence.

Scan the QR code to access the link to download your bonuses!

Printed in Great Britain
by Amazon